# AWAKEN
## YOUR SLEEP

Cultivate Your Sleep Friendship for Restful Nights

EXPANDED EDITION
includes
*The Sleep Alchemist*

*Bibi Ohlsson*

www.bibiohlsson.com

Awaken Your Sleep is a revitalized version of How to Build a Robust Relationship with Sleep (Bibi Ohlsson, 2023), and is available in wiro-o binding (978-82-845-1073-6) as well as epub (9788284511955)

This softcover edition you're holding is an upcycled and expanded second edition that delves deeper into the world of sleep, offering effective and practical strategies to transform your sleep habits. A new section, "The Sleep Alchemist," introduces an enchanting approach to cultivating restorative rest.

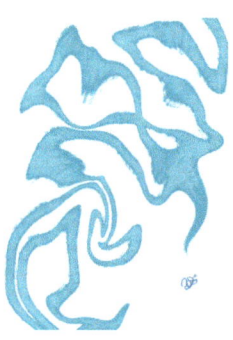

Disclaimer: Your Sleep Matters

While this book is full of helpful sleep information,
it's not meant to replace professional medical advice.
Think of it as a tool alongside your physician's guidance!

*Even when sleep feels untouchable,*
*each sunrise boldly proclaims*
*the promise of a fresh start.*

*Like the albatross*
*gracefully sleeping mid-flight,*
*you possess the potential to adapt,*
*a quiet resilience.*

*Believe you can*
*nurture your resilience*
*and weave rest into your life skillfully,*
*finding the restorative power of sleep*
*even amid the bustle of your days.*

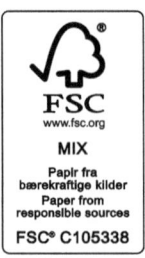

Copyediting: Grammarly.
Illustrations:  Canva. Bibi Ohlsson
Publisher: BoD - Books on Demand, Oslo, Norway
Printing: BoD - Books on Demand, Norderstedt, Tyskland

ISBN: 978-82-845-1093-4

# Table of Content:

# Table of Content - cont'

# Foreword

My passion - and purpose - is helping people bring out the best version of themselves. As a positive psychology coach, I've seen how focusing and building on what comes naturally and works well, the core and character strengths, can lead to incredible transformations.

That's my motivation for creating a sleep guide – to help awaken your sleep and unlock the hidden superpower of rest!

Think about it: getting enough sleep makes us more patient, focused, energized, and healthier.

Not only does this improve our own lives, it ripples outward. Rested people build happier families, stronger communities, and ultimately, a kinder world.

My hope is this guide empowers you to change your mindset around sleep, rewrite stressful thoughts, and approach bedtime with optimism.

Here's to discovering a world where rest is not a luxury, but an essential pillar of your vibrant, joyful life.

Warmly,
*Bibi*

*Uncover the Secrets of Your Sleep*

# Awaken Your Sleep Power

# Discover Your Hidden Sleep World

Picture sleep as a vast, unexplored territory within your own body. A hidden world you visit each night, shaping your energy, mood, and well-being in ways you might not fully understand. It's time to embark on a journey of discovery!

**Unraveling the Secrets:** Forget the idea of sleep as simply being "off." While you rest, incredible things happen – your brain strengthens memories, your body repairs itself, and your emotional landscape resets.

**The Evolution of Rest:** Sleep changes throughout life. Understanding where you are now—your patterns, your struggles—is the first step towards making sleep work for you in this phase of your life.

**The Nurturing Factor:** Like any meaningful relationship, your connection with sleep thrives on attention and care. Cultivating a calming evening unwind is a powerful way to demonstrate that care. It's also crucial to understand your emotions, thoughts, and environment – all of which play a crucial role in shaping your sleep experience.

# Decoding Your Sleep Signals

Like a close friend, your body has a unique way of communicating its needs.

Understanding sleep's subtle language is vital to building a solid foundation for your sleep friendship.

Many people think yawning is the only sign of tiredness. Still, your body actually starts sending out signals long before that point.

Irritability, difficulty concentrating, and even increased hunger can be early hints that you're starting to run low on sleep.

Here's how some people describe those subtle sleep signals:

"I get irritable and crave late afternoon snacks. That might be a sign of sleepiness."

"I'm scrolling mindlessly through social media, not really engaged in anything"

"I'm starting to see a pattern between restless nights and days when I skipped my morning walk."

"I feel colder than usual, like I need an extra layer even when the temperature hasn't changed."

"I feel more sensitive than normal, and little things easily get under my skin."

**Taking Action:** The key is not just respecting the sleep signals but understanding their benefits. By taking short breaks for mental recharge or incorporating calming activities like mindfulness into your day, you're not just responding thoughtfully; your body is also paving the way for a more restful sleep. This understanding empowers you, giving you the tools to take control of your sleep and overall well-being.

**The Result:** By attuning to your body's natural rhythms and giving priority to quality sleep, you foster a healthier sleep routine and strengthen the foundation of your overall well-being. This heightened awareness is not just a source of optimism; it empowers you to take intentional steps toward achieving the deep, restorative sleep that you rightfully deserve. This positive shift in your sleep habits can lead to a more vibrant and satisfying life.

What are the sensations and sleep signals associated with your need for sleep?

How can you better respect your body's sleep cues and act accordingly?

# Outsmart the Sleep Struggle

Remember those carefree nights when you quickly melted into sleep? Now, something's changed. The harder you chase sleep, the more it slips through your fingers. Welcome to the frustrating world of sleep struggles! But here's the good news: there's a path out of this trap.

## Challenging the Myths

It appears you're putting a lot of effort into solving your sleep issues, and that's admirable. However, there's a common mistake that many people make when trying to fall asleep. Trying to force sleep might not be the best approach. Demanding, "I must sleep now!" puts your body into a state of anxiety, making everything worse.

It's similar to the "don't think of a pink elephant" problem - the more you try not to think about it, the more it pops up. Similarly, the more you try to force yourself to sleep, the harder it becomes to fall asleep.

Frustration mounts, pillows get tossed, and nights become battle-grounds. This isn't the way sleep is supposed to be. If struggle defines your relationship with sleep, a fresh approach is needed.

## Finding the Gentle Path

The secret to better sleep often lies in doing less – less striving, less worrying. It's similar to cultivating a friendship – understanding and ease are essential, not forceful tactics.

Your sleep journey is unique, filled with personal habits, worries, and even those odd thoughts that seem to pop up when you turn out the light. Why don't we explore these together!

Sleep struggles I want to outsmart:

## Beyond the Basics

Yes, catching up on sleep over the weekend helps, but research shows you can't fully erase sleep debt that way. Shifting sleep patterns between weekdays and weekends can lead to social jet lag! Consistency is crucial for your internal clock. How about trying a daily early afternoon power nap instead?

Waking up during the night is normal, and brief awakenings shouldn't make you feel like a "bad sleeper." What matters is if you can fall asleep again quickly. Instead of reaching for your phone to check the time, try some breathing exercises to signal to your body that it's safe to drift back off.

While some people still swear by the 20-minute rule (if you can't fall asleep within 20 minutes, get out of bed), it can have drawbacks, especially for insomniacs. Up to date sleep advice often recommends staying in bed and trying relaxation techniques to avoid negative associations with sleep space.

Lastly, that early afternoon slump isn't laziness! It's a natural dip in your body's energy levels. Hydrate and take a brisk walk for a boost, or consider a short power nap if possible.

Outsmarting the sleep struggle can help you move from frustration to feeling empowered. Remember, the key isn't brute force but a gentle understanding of your unique sleep patterns.

Think of it as detective work. Your daily routines and habits contain hidden clues that can reveal your natural tendencies toward sleep. This awareness can help you harness your inner strengths to create a sleep routine that works for you.

Actions I must take to outsmart my sleep struggles:

# Harness Your Natural Abilities

Your strengths are the core of who you are—the things you do best and come naturally to you. Using those innate abilities, you can unlock your potential to overcome sleep challenges and create the restful life you deserve.

## Consider these questions to guide you on your sleep journey to improve your sleep:

How can you leverage your self-regultaion to establish consitent sleep patterns and create relaxing pre-sleep rituals that work for you?

What intriguing ways can your natural problem-solving abilities help you identify the root causes of your sleep struggles and find personalized solutions that resonate with you?

How can you harness your resilience to stay committed and keep going, especially when progress feels slow?

Take a moment to consider how you can enhance your sleep by focusing on these aspects of yourself.

**Self-Leadership:**
How can you personally take charge of improving your sleep health, and what specific actions can you take to initiate positive changes in this area?

How can you hold yourself accountable for maintaining healthy sleep habits, and what strategies can you use to stay on track with your sleep goals?

**Self-Determination:**
What motivates you to pursue change and adopt new sleep patterns?

How can you strengthen your commitment to embracing change concerning your sleep habits?

**Self-Care:**
Some people find that making self-care a non-negotiable part of their routine by honoring the profound significance of getting good rest is helpful.

How can you prioritize quality sleep as essential to your overall well-being? Remember, by prioritizing your sleep, you prioritize your health and self-care.

# Tame Your Sleep Thoughts

Sometimes, our thoughts are the biggest obstacles to a good night's rest.

Have you ever found yourself awake with these thoughts running through your head?

> "I'm never going to fall asleep!"
> "If I don't sleep enough tonight, tomorrow will be awful."
> "I should just give up and get out of bed."

These negative and often exaggerated thoughts create anxiety and fuel your sleeplessness.

What common negative or unhelpful thoughts
keep you up at night?

What patterns or triggers have you noticed
that lead to these thoughts?

How do you typically react to these thoughts?

Here's the good news: you can learn to challenge
and reframe these unhelpful sleep thoughts.

# Neutralize Sleep Worries

**Notice:**
Start paying attention to your bedtime thought patterns. What messages are you telling yourself about sleep?

**Ask:**
Are They True? Do you have evidence to support these thoughts, or are they based on fear and frustration? Often, they're not realistic.

**Reframe with Kindness:**
Replace those negative thoughts with more balanced and helpful ones. For example, instead of "I'm never going to fall asleep!" think, "My body knows how to rest, and it may take a little time tonight."

**Acknowledge** that you're able to master realistic thinking. By shifting your mindset, you give yourself a calmer bedtime experience.

*Negative thought:*

*"My heart is racing, and my stress level is high.*
*I'm never going to be able to fall asleep with this feeling."*

*Reframing with kindness:*

*"I'm feeling anxious right now, but I know this sensation will pass.*
*I'm going to focus on taking deep breaths and relaxing my body.*
*This will help me feel calmer and at ease,*
*allowing me to fall asleep naturally."*

# Nurture Your Sleep Friendship

Have you ever considered sleep a vital relationship? To experience its benefits, it needs time and attention.

A helpful tip is to draw upon the wisdom we've gained in other meaningful relationships to guide us:

**Teamwork Mentality:** Approach sleep as your ally, not your enemy. Instead of fighting it, work with it to achieve better rest and overall well-being.

**Patience and Understanding:** Change rarely happens overnight. Be kind to yourself as you create new sleep habits. Celebrate even small steps forward, knowing they add up to lasting improvement.

**Focus on the Positive:** Dwelling on challenging nights only creates more anxiety. Instead, acknowledge those nights and shift your focus. Celebrate the good nights and tell yourself, "Tonight is a new opportunity to wake up rested."

**Challenge and Reframe:** When unhelpful thoughts like "I'll never sleep well again" creep in, don't let them linger. Reframe them: "This is challenging right now, but I'm learning new skills, and things will improve."

**Acknowledge and Appreciate:** Recognize the benefits you experience on nights when sleep comes easily. This reinforces positive experiences.

**Sustaining Motivation:** Remind yourself how sleep affects your mood, energy, and productivity. This keeps you motivated as you build your sleep friendship.

With consistency and a commitment to
working together, you and sleep
can transform your relationship
from a source of struggle
into a foundation for lasting well-being.

# Design Your Sleep Blueprint

The journey to better sleep begins with honest self-assessment. Reflecting on your current habits, beliefs, and environment reveals valuable insights about what might hold you back. This self-awareness empowers you to take charge of your sleep journey, fostering autonomy and healthy self-leadership. And these insights are the foundation for building the sleep you crave.

## Neglect and the Need for Change

Our fast-paced lives often lead to unconsciously neglecting sleep. However, consistent sleep deprivation has ripple effects on our physical and mental well-being. Conversely, prioritizing sleep revitalizes our energy, improves our mood, and enhances our overall quality of life.

> In what ways might my current habits be impacting my sleep quality?
>
> How could better sleep quality transform my energy levels, mood, and overall well-being?
>
> What am I willing to change or prioritize to create a healthier connection to sleep?

## Space and Respect

The concept of rest goes beyond sleeping. Do you view rest as an indulgence or a necessity? Transforming your sleep starts with respecting its importance and creating a space that honors your need for rejuvenation. Shifting your beliefs about rest can lead to a more fulfilling sleep experience.

What are my beliefs about rest, and how can I shift those to support my well-being?

What changes to my bedroom would invite relaxation and better sleep?

Which routines, habits, or thoughts might sabotage my rest, and how can I manage them?

## Presence vs. Distraction

Transitioning to sleep mode can be challenging in today's world of constant stimulation. A mindful wind-down routine signals to your brain and body that it's time to rest, creating a smoother path to falling asleep. Conversely, remaining plugged into distractions throughout the evening can leave your mind racing, making sleep elusive.

What would an ideal wind-down routine look and feel like for me?

How can I establish a clear boundary between my waking life and wind-down routine?

## Compromise and Shared Space

Whether you share your sleep space with a partner, children, or furry friends, finding balance is crucial. Open communication and minor adjustments can create an environment where everyone's sleep needs are respected. Conversely, ignoring your sleep environment or the needs of those you share it with can lead to fragmented rest and frustration for all involved.

> What adjustments to my sleep environment could promote greater comfort and relaxation?
>
> How can I balance my needs and those of my sleeping partners for optimal rest?

## Consistency and Progress

While quick fixes are tempting, sustainable sleep improvement requires consistency and patience. Designing a sleep schedule that works for you and celebrating small victories keeps you motivated and moving toward restful nights. On the other hand, erratic sleep patterns can throw your body's rhythms out of sync, making it challenging to fall asleep and stay asleep.

> How can I build a sleep schedule that meets my life's demands while prioritizing rest?
>
> What milestones and victories, no matter how small, will I acknowledge and celebrate along the way?
>
> What support systems, tools, or strategies will help me tay on track with my sleep goals?

# Befriend Your Sleep Needs

It's time to move from awareness to action! What you've read sets the stage, but the transformation happens only when you apply it!

Think of this book as your hands-on sleep improvement workbook. As you work through it, I encourage you to:

**Crafting Your Sleep Playbook:** What if you make this guide your personal sleep-guide to crafting a sleep experience that supports your well-being? You'll gain valuable self-knowledge as you answer questions, track your journey, and reflect on insights. This empowers you to embrace healthy self-leadership on your path to better rest.

**Revisit and Revise:** Your understanding of sleep will deepen as you continue reading. Return to these earlier sections periodically. You might be surprised how your answers and thoughts evolve!

**Celebrate Your Growth:** Acknowledging big and small wins is crucial for staying motivated. Your journal is the perfect place to record your progress.

Remember, a stronger relationship with sleep isn't built overnight. It takes consistency, effort, and a willingness to learn and adjust. But the results – feeling rested, energized,and ready for each new day– will be more than worth it!

Reading something is great, and it is even better when you also
internalize the information and make it your own.
Take note of what it inspires in you so you can refer back to it later.

Start doing:

Stop doing:

Do more of:

Do less of:

*Tonight Could Be the Night*
# Every Night Holds Potential

# Building an Unbreakable Bond

Think of sleep as the bedrock upon which your day is built. You feel more stable, focused, and healthier when you consistently get enough quality rest. On the other hand, without a solid foundation, everything else in life—your mood, performance, relationships—start to crumble.

Sometimes, 'Tonight Could Be the Night!' feels impossible. When insomnia drags on, it's easy to lose hope. But even amidst the most challenging nights, the potential exists.

We all have nights that don't go as planned. Instead of labeling them 'bad, ' consider them opportunities. What can you learn about your sleep patterns from a challenging night? That knowledge is power! You might want to explore how to shift your mindset and build habits that create fertile ground for restful nights to take root.

Sleep can feel elusive, especially if you struggle with it consistently. But rest assured, you have the innate potential to power up and build a healthier relationship with sleep.

While understanding sleep science can be helpful, the connection – the friendship – unlocks more restful nights. You'll gradually improve your energy and well-being by knowing your sleep needs and cultivating healthy habits.

Like building any strong bond, your friendship with sleep requires effort, commitment, and understanding. And the rewards of a good night's rest? They're more than worth the investment!

# Understand the Power of Sleep

We instinctively know sleep is essential, but its transformative impact extends beyond simply feeling rested. Let's uncover the fascinating processes happening within your body and brain during those restorative hours:

**Energy Restoration:** Imagine sleep as your internal power station. It replenishes your depleted physical and mental energy stores, leaving you feeling revitalized and ready to face the day.

**Memory Consolidation:** Sleep is your brain's librarian, diligently organizing and storing the day's experiences. This strengthens memories, transforming them into lasting knowledge and skills that benefit you long-term.

**Immune System Boost:** Sleep is your body's defense system's best friend. It provides critical support, allowing your body to effectively fight off illness and maintain optimal health.

**Emotional Regulation:** Quality sleep acts like a reset button for emotions. It helps regulate moods, reduces stress levels, and promotes greater well-being.

# The Science Behind Restful Nights

Sleep isn't a single, static state; it's a dynamic journey.
You cycle through different stages – Light Sleep, Deep Sleep, and REM –
each offering unique benefits.

Think of these cycles as laps around a track. About 5-6 laps (cycles) are
needed for optimal restfulness. Deep sleep is the most restorative, aiding
physical repair, memory consolidation, and immune function.

**Timing Your Sleep Cycle:** A little reverse engineering helps ensure you
get those crucial deep sleep cycles! Most people need around 450 minutes (7.5 hours) of sleep. If you want to wake up at 6:30 AM, count back
those 450 minutes, meaning you'd need to be asleep by 11:00 PM. Of
course, this is a guideline, and remember to include the time it takes to
fall asleep.

Understanding this symphony of processes
while you slumber reveals how deeply sleep affects
your overall well-being.

But it's not just about the science; it's also about
listening to your internal conversation about sleep.
Is that dialogue supportive, or does it create
obstacles to restful nights?

Consider how your thoughts and self-talk
influence your sleep experience.

# Seek a Connection with Sleep

Sometimes, even our strongest bonds go through rough patches. Work demands, worries, and body changes can strain our connection with sleep. But that doesn't mean the relationship is beyond repair. You can mend this vital friendship with understanding and effort from both sides.

It might be time to listen to the part of yourself that's desperate for rest.

Here's a message from that exhausted place:

*Dear Sleep,*

*I miss you terribly. We used to be inseparable, but lately, we barely speak. Tossing, turning, racing thoughts – peaceful nights seem like distant memories. Can we go back to how things were? I'm ready to do whatever it takes to mend our friendship.*

*Desperately Yours,*
*Me*

If you could write a letter to Sleep, what would you say?

What do you miss most about a good night's rest?

How has a strained relationship with sleep impacted your life?

A flicker of hope stirs within you. Sleep has heard your plea. Is there an answer echoing back?

*Dearest Me,*

*I know things haven't been easy. Believe me, I miss you too. But our friendship isn't just about me showing up. We have to work as a team.*
*Are you ready to make some changes – your routines, your bedroom, even some of those thoughts that keep you up at night?*
*If so, we can make this work.*

*Always Here for You,*
*Sleep*

What changes are you willing to make to improve your sleep?

How might those changes help strengthen your bond with sleep?

What if you could improve your waking life and discover the benefits of sleep by nurturing a healthy sleep friendship and mastering sleep's hidden control panel?

# Your Inner Dialogue

Imagine having a much-needed internal conversation. It's not about blame but gaining honest insight. Here's how that dialogue might unfold...

**You:** I'm exhausted and frustrated. Sleep has become another battle I'm losing. My mind races, my body won't cooperate, and I resent the concept.

**Inner Wisdom:** It's understandable. Relentlessly pushing yourself and expecting your body to switch off will create tension. But resentment won't solve the problem.

**You:** I know. But it's hard to break the cycle. There's always too much to do and too much to worry about. I feel like I'm running on empty.

**Inner Wisdom:** That's precisely why sleep is critical. It's your chance to recharge, to give your body and mind the restoration they crave. Denying yourself rest actually makes it harder to handle those challenges.

**You:** You're right. But how do I make the change? I've tried all the usual tips, and nothing seems to stick.

**Inner Wisdom:** The issue might not be the tips themselves but how you approach them. It's easy to fall into an all-or-nothing mindset. Remember, developing a healthy relationship with sleep is a journey, not a destination.

**You:** I see. I do get easily discouraged. If sleep isn't perfect, I feel like a failure.

**Inner Wisdom:** That's a common trap. Try focusing on the effort, not just the outcome. Appreciate the nights you stick to your routine, even if sleep is elusive. Celebrate the small wins - like waking up consistently or being more mindful of your sleep habits. That's real progress!

**You:** I like focusing on the effort, not just the results. Speaking of effort, where do I even start? There's so much information about sleep out there; it's overwhelming.

**Inner Wisdom:** Shall we break it down? At its core, good sleep hygiene is about consistency and creating a conducive environment for rest. Could we start with your sleep schedule?

**You:** That does seem like an excellent place to begin. I'm terrible about having a consistent bedtime.

**Inner Wisdom:** That's okay! Knowing where you struggle is the first step. Think about a realistic bedtime that gets you the rest you need. Then, the real challenge is sticking to it, even on weekends. Your body's internal clock thrives on regularity.

**You:** Okay, I'll choose a target bedtime. But what about winding down before bed? My mind races the moment I get into bed.

**Inner Wisdom:** A calming evening unwind is crucial. Experiment to discover what works for you. A warm bath or shower, gentle stretches, or reading a relaxing book can signal to your brain that it's time to transition away from the day's stresses.

**You:** Is using my phone to read before bed okay, or is that a bad habit?

**Inner Wisdom:** Ideally, you want to minimize screen time right before bed. Devices' blue light can suppress melatonin production, making it harder to fall asleep. A physical book, or even a relaxing audiobook, would be softer on your eyes and brain. Reading can also help slow your thoughts and prepare you for sleep.

**You:** Interesting. Is there anything else about sleep science that I should be aware of? It all feels a bit mysterious.

**Inner Wisdom:** Absolutely! Sleep is incredibly complex, and researchers are constantly learning new things. One important concept is sleep cycles. Throughout the night, you cycle through different stages of sleep, each with a distinct purpose.

**You:** Tell me more!

**Inner Wisdom:** Think of your sleep as a nighttime journey with several stops. These 'stops' are your sleep cycles. Each cycle has a different purpose:

- Light Sleep: You're drifting off, so waking up is easy.
- Deep Sleep: This is the good stuff! Your body repairs, the immune system boosts, and the brain files away memories.
- REM Sleep: Dreamland! Your brain is very active, processing emotions and making connections between ideas.

Imagine each sleep cycle is like a lap around a track. You start with a light warm-up (light sleep), then really get going (deep sleep), followed by a mental cool-down (REM). You need several complete 'laps' to feel your best!

**You:** Wow, I had no idea there was so much going on! Based on these sleep cycles, is there a way to optimize my wake-up timing?

**Inner Wisdom:** Absolutely! Remember, those sleep cycles last roughly 90 minutes each. The trick is waking up at the end of a cycle rather than in the middle. For instance, waking up during deep sleep can leave you dizzy and disoriented.

**You:** That makes sense. But how do I put that into practice?

**Inner Wisdom:** How about some reverse engineering? Say you want to wake up at 6:30 AM. Aim to be asleep by 11:00 PM to feel most refreshed, allowing five complete sleep cycles. Of course, you might need to adjust slightly depending on how long you fall asleep.

**You:** That's incredibly helpful! I'm going to experiment with this right away.

**Inner Wisdom:** That's great! Tracking your sleep patterns can also provide valuable insights. Note how you feel when you wake up at different times, and you can fine-tune your ideal sleep schedule.

# Level Up Your Sleep Game

You've mastered the sleep basics; now it's time to improve your sleep strategy. Experimenting with powerful techniques can help you sleep more soundly and enhance your overall well-being.

## Harness the Power of Your Day

Your daytime habits profoundly impact the quality of your nighttime rest. Here are some simple but effective ways to optimize your day for better sleep:

**Hydration:** Dehydration can cause fatigue and reduce cognitive function. Drink enough water throughout the day to stay hydrated and alert.

**Midday Movement Reset:** If you work a sedentary job, short breaks for movement (e.g., a quick walk or simple stretches) can work wonders for your energy levels and evening relaxation.

**The Coffee Power Nap** might sound surprising, but it works for many people! Experiment with a short nap (20-30 minutes) right after a coffee, ideally early to mid-afternoon.

**After-Dinner Stroll:** A gentle walk after dinner does more than aid digestion. It signals to your body and mind that the active part of your day is winding down.

## Master Your Light Exposure

Light acts as the primary cue for your body's sleep-wake cycle. Strategically managing your light exposure throughout the day can significantly improve sleep quality.

**Morning Sunshine:** Exposure to morning sunlight helps synchronize your internal clock, promoting alertness during the day and making it easier to fall asleep at night.

**Evening Dim-Down:** Dim the lights and minimize screen time (with its disruptive blue light) at least an hour before bed. This signals your brain that it's time to wind down and encourages the natural production of melatonin, your sleep hormone.

What else? How can you better master your light exposure?

# Optimize Your Sleep Environment

Your sleep environment plays a remarkable role in how well you rest. Here are a few simple adjustments that can make a big difference:

**Tidiness:** Keeping your bedroom clean and tidy can help reduce stress and promote a sense of calm. Make your bed every morning, clear clutter from surfaces, and create a space that feels calm and organized. A tidy room can help you feel more relaxed and ready for sleep.

**Blackout Curtains:** Light can disrupt your circadian rhythm and make it harder to fall asleep. Blackout curtains can help block out light from outside and create a dark environment conducive to sleep.

**Plants:** Bringing plants into your bedroom can help purify the air and create a calming atmosphere. Some plants, such as lavender, jasmine, gardenia, rosemary, and aloe vera, are also known for their soothing properties, which can help promote relaxation.

**Weighted Blankets:** For some people, a weighted blanket's deep pressure stimulation provides a calming, comforting sensation that can reduce anxiety and promote relaxation. Choose a blanket that's about 10% of your body weight.

**Cool It Down:** A slightly cooler room (around 60-67 degrees F / 16-20 degrees C) mimics your body's natural temperature drop as you prepare for sleep, making it easier to fall asleep and stay asleep throughout the night.

**Eliminate Noise:** Noise is one of the most common causes of sleep disturbance. Use earplugs or a white noise machine to block out noise from the outside world and create a quiet sleep environment.

## Mindful Techniques for Restful Nights

Establishing a calming bedtime routine can help you relax, reduce stress, and promote restful sleep. These techniques are simple yet effective and can significantly improve sleep quality.

**Avoid Late-Night Snacking:** Eating late at night can disrupt your body's natural digestive process and interfere with sleep. Avoid heavy meals or snacks closer than a few hours to bedtime, and opt for lighter options if you need a snack.

> **Core Temperature Rhythm:** Our body temperature naturally drops at bedtime, aiding sleepiness. A cool shower in the evening mimics this natural drop, sending your body the right signal.

> **Post-Shower Warm-Up:** The contrast between the cool shower and the subsequent warming up promotes relaxation and prepares the body for sleep.

**Find Your Sonic Bliss:** Pink noise, white noise, rain sounds...the options are endless. These steady, soothing sounds can block distractions and lull you into deep relaxation.

**Tense, Then Release:** Progressive muscle relaxation is like a stress-buster for your whole body. Tense and release different muscle groups, guiding your focus away from worries and towards physical sensations.

**Mindfulness Meditation:** Sit or lie comfortably, close your eyes, and focus on your breath. If your mind starts to wander, gently bring it back to your breath. Do this for a few minutes daily to start seeing the benefits.

**Breathwork for Calm:** Deep breathing exercises can quiet a racing mind and ease your body into a state of relaxation.

Try the "4-8" technique

Mindfully inhale through your nose for a count of 4.
With awareness, exhale through your nose for a count of 8.
Repeat for several minutes, focusing entirely on your breath

Start doing:

## You Are in Control

The journey to better sleep takes time and practice. There will be set-backs, but don't get discouraged!  Understanding your sleep-sabotaging behaviours is key:

**Tune in:** Before reaching for your phone late at night or skipping your evening walk, pause. Are you feeling bored, stressed, or anxious?

**Choose Your Response:** You have a choice once you identfy the trigger. Instead of giving in to old habits, select a technique from your sleep toolkit. If you're stressed, try deep breathing. If you're feeling restless, a warm shower could do the trick.

Remember, you are the expert on yourself!  With self-awareness and practice, you can transform your sleep.

Celebrate those wins - even small changes are a sign you're on the right track!

# Ignite Hope for Better Sleep

Did you know that feeling hopeful can pave the way for better sleep? Hope reduces stress, lifts your mood, and creates the perfect conditions for restful nights. It's a win-win!

## Hope Has Two Powerful Sides

Hope isn't just wishful thinking. It has two essential aspects:

**Hope as a Feeling:** The deep-seated belief that better sleep is possible.

**Hope as an Action:** Taking practical steps to build the better future you envision.

Hope might feel abstract, but it's the catalyst for positive change in sleep. Believing that better sleep is possible motivates you to try those new techniques, stick with your evening routine even when you're tired, and track your progress.

Want to take those hopeful feelings and turn them into action to transform your sleep?

## Hope in Action: Reclaim Your Rest

**Imagine this:** You've battled poor sleep for ages. You start consistently using a relaxation technique before bed and finally drift off more easily. How does it feel?

Let yourself experience those positive emotions, and let that feeling fuel your determination to try the following:

**Feel the Hope:** Instead of dwelling on your struggles, picture yourself waking up refreshed.

Have you woken up refreshed after following a simple yet calming pre-bed ritual?

**Act on Hope:** What actions can bridge the gap between where you are now and those restful nights you crave?  Maybe it's a worry-reframing technique to address a stressful thought pattern that keeps you awake.

## Hope Needs Backup

We all have those nights – TV wins out over sleep, scrolling steals precious minutes, and negative thoughts whisper, "You'll never fall asleep anyway." This throws off your sleep rhythm and makes relaxation harder.

## The Solution?

- Recognize those sabotaging moments.
- Have a plan to get back on track with your evening unwind.

Remember, hope is the bridge that connects you to more restful sleep. Every effort you make, whether creating a relaxing pre-bed routine or simply believing in the possibility of better sleep, strengthens your bond with sleeping.

As your friendship with sleep grows more robust, you'll have more of the restful nights, which you crave.

# Your Sleep Superpower

A grateful heart leads to a sleepy heart! Try this before bed:

**Two New Things:**
What are two new things you learned today? Even small wins count!

**Celebrate Yourself:**
What are two things you did well today? No victory is too small.

**Savor the Good:**
What two things brought you joy today?

**The Bottom Line:**
Hope and sleep are a powerful team.
By actively believing in your ability
to create change and taking simple steps forward,
you'll create a positive cycle of rest and optimism.

# Navigate Your Sleep Journey

**The One-Change Challenge:**
Choose one specific action to enhance your evening unwind this week.
Small and consistent is vital — what's your first step?

**Practice Self-Compassion:**
Bad nights happen. Instead of beating yourself up, try this: What's one
supportive, encouraging thing you can say to yourself about your sleep
journey?

Do more of:

# Rethink Your Sleep Struggles

Setbacks are normal.

Instead of "Ugh, I'm back to square one!" ask yourself: What can I learn from this experience to use next time?

**Negative Thought:** "I'll never get back to sleep if I wake up now."

**Reframe:** "This is temporary. I can use a relaxation technique and drift off again."

**Negative Thought:** "Everyone else sleeps fine. I'm the only one struggling."

**Reframe:** "Sleep issues are common. I'm not alone, and there are solutions."

**Negative Thought:** "If I don't get 8 hours, my day is ruined."

**Reframe:** "Every bit of sleep helps. Even if it's less than ideal, I can still function."

# Questions to Spark Positivity

Transforming your sleep is a marathon, not a sprint. Take a moment to appreciate all your steps, big or small. This isn't about perfection; it's about progress!

**Awareness:**
What have you learned about yourself and your sleep habits that you didn't know before?

**Small Victories:**
Did you even have one night when you fell asleep a little easier this week? Or did you try a technique that helped?

**Shifting Mindset:**
Have you noticed your inner voice becoming kinder towards your sleep struggles?

**Staying Motivated:**
What's the one thing that excites you most about improving your sleep?

# Escape Your Sleep Illusion

In the relentless pursuit of success, we often believe that sacrificing sleep equals higher productivity. In reality, sleep deprivation undermines your true potential. Here's a glimpse into the costs of running on empty:

**Brain Drain:** Your sharp mind becomes clouded by mental fog, making complex problems seem impossible and decisions feel impulsive.

**Energy Crisis:** You're surviving, not thriving. Caffeinated and worn out, you lose the joy and drive for sustained effort.

**Stress Monster:** Lack of sleep weakens resilience and hijacks emotional control, making one less adaptable to inevitable challenges.

Do less of:

## Boost Your Performance

It's time for a strategic shift if constant fatigue holds you back. Forget the latest life hacks – sleep is your secret weapon for peak performance. Imagine this:

**Work smarter, not harder:** Deep rest unlocks a creative, focused mind capable of brilliant solutions and efficient execution.

**Make better, faster decisions:** Say goodbye to foggy judgment. Sleep brings clarity and confidence for bold action.

**Bring your A-game consistently:** Quality sleep is your fuel for sustained energy, unflinching focus, and the resilience to push through any obstacle.

What's one crucial task your ambition depends on but mental fatigue always seems to derail?

How would laser-sharp focus and relentless energy transform your ability to achieve that goal?

## Your Secret To Success

Have you ever wondered how high potentials maintain energy, focus, and drive? Talent is not the only thing that sets them apart.

Sleep is a critical part of their success strategy, powering their ability to:

- Maintain razor-sharp focus on complex problems.
- Fuel the relentless pursuit of goals with sustained energy.
- Remain calm, collected, and resilient amidst setbacks.

What if the same secret [sleep] could fuel your journey to the success you want?

## Build Your Sleep-Powered Success

Sleep's benefits aren't just a feeling – they're rooted in incredible transformations happening while you rest:

**Memory Masterclass:** Reinforce knowledge and skills, turning experiences into mastery.

**Brain Detox:** Clear away mental clutter, restoring cognitive clarity and preventing long-term damage.

**Stress Buster:** Reset stress hormones, allowing you to tackle any challenge calmly.

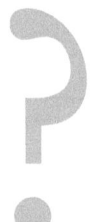

What if every night of rest could make you sharper, stronger,and more resilient for the challenges ahead?

## Reclaim Your Edge

It's time to shift the narrative – sleep isn't a luxury; it's a necessity! Here's how to prioritize peak performance:

**The Power of Routine:** Consistent bedtimes and wake-up times (even on weekends!) optimize your sleep cycles.

**Your Sleep Sanctuary:** A dimly lit, quiet room with a calming bedtime routine signals to your brain that it's time to relax.

**Gift Yourself Rest:** Treat sleep like a crucial appointment. You wouldn't skip an important client meeting!

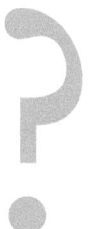

What if you could reclaim your competitive edge simply by changing your relationship with sleep?

## Conquer Your Ambitions

This isn't about adding to your workload but working smarter, not harder. Imagine yourself effortlessly crushing a complex project thanks to a well-rested, clear-thinking mind. That's the advantage you gain with sleep as your ally.

Sleep powers your ambition. It's your investment in a future where you achieve your biggest dreams with clarity, energy, and unwavering determination.

## Ask Yourself:

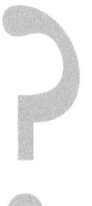

What extraordinary outcome could better sleep make possible for you?

What's the first small step you'll take tonight to improve your sleep?

The stories of how others have harnessed this sleep superpower can be inspiring.

It's time to introduce you to a few individuals who found success unexpectedly thanks to a renewed relationship with sleep.

# Meet Some Sleepers

Our sleep experiences are as unique as we are. These relatable stories show that if others can overcome challenges and find better sleep, so can you!

**Gina: The Sleep Enthusiast:** "Sleep is my superpower! Consistent evening unwinding keeps me feeling great and crushing my to-do list."

**Gabrielle: The Accidental Napper:** "Sometimes a quick nap hits the reset button better than anything else."

**Shelly: Light Sleeper, Deep Thinker:** "I've learned to roll with those wake-ups. A little reading or meditation, and I'm back to sleep."

**Mark: The Midnight Writer:** "I'm wired for late-night creativity. Finding a flexible work schedule was a game-changer."

**The Relentless CEO Sarah:** "I thrive on adrenaline, but even I'm hitting burnout. How do I slow down without sabotaging my career?"
Sarah was used to conquering challenges through sheer force of will. Learning to prioritize rest felt counterintuitive. But even small changes, like 20-minute nature walks or brief meditation sessions, helped shift her overactive mindset and create space for pre-bed relaxation. She discovered that rest wasn't a sign of weakness but a strategic tool for sustainable success.

**Henry, the Adaptable Entrepreneur:** "My business and family always come first, and sleep is always last. I seem to get by on less than most, but I'm reaching my limit. What's a sustainable solution?"

Henry didn't crumble easily, but constant sleep deprivation wore him down. He learned that it's not just about the quantity of sleep but the quality. By optimizing his sleep environment, developing a quick "power down" routine, and being strategic about when Henry could catch up on rest, Henry managed to function at a high level even without the ideal 8 hours. While he still longed for more consistent rest, he found a way to make his unique sleep needs work within his busy life.

As you continue on your journey towards a better night's rest, it's important to remember that sleep isn't just about feeling refreshed in the morning. It's about nurturing a lifelong bond with your body and mind. You're investing in your well-being and growth by embracing sleep and committing to healthy sleep habits.

Close your eyes briefly and imagine a world dedicated to restful nights and wakeful days!

Reading something is great, and it is even better when you also internalize the information and make it your own. Take note of what it inspires in you so you can refer back to it later.

What are your thoughts on the potential connection between sleep difficulties that could signify that you're holding onto old thought patterns and behaviors that no longer serve you?

How do you think engaging in sleep-interfering behaviors, such as excessive worry or screen time before bed, might be fueled by an underlying resistance to change and growth?

How might specific thoughts or beliefs about sleep, yourself, or your life might influence your sleep patterns?

What unresolved emotional issues or past traumas might be surfacing at night and disrupting your sleep?

In what way do you believe reframing your thoughts about sleep and your wakeful life creates a more optimistic and empowering mindset?

*Nurture the Bond for Deeper Rest*

# The Friendship You Didn't Know You Needed

# The Value of Friendship

Think about your closest friendships. Some start with a spark—you just click with someone instantly. Others blossom over time as you discover shared interests, vulnerabilities, and the joy of mutual support.

Nurturing friendships enriches our lives and helps us grow as individuals. But have you ever considered the possibility of a unique, life-changing friendship with sleep?

# Reframe Your Sleep Mindset

One approach to improving your relationship with sleep is to change the way you think about it.

For instance, instead of fixating on the challenge of falling asleep, you could reframe this as a journey of learning to sleep better, a path that holds the promise of growth and improvement.

By consistently applying new strategies and being patient with yourself, you can pave the way for a healthier and more positive relationship with sleep.

Take a moment to reflect on your current approach to falling asleep. How can you reframe it to foster a more positive and productive mindset, actively engaging in the process of change?

# Be Kind & Understanding

It's important to remember that facing challenges with sleep is a common part of life. Acknowledging this is the first step towards finding a solution. Seeking assistance or aiming for improvement is a commendable decision. It requires courage to prioritize your own well-being. Be compassionate to yourself throughout this process.

Experiencing a night of restlessness is not a sign of failure – it's a natural part of being human. Instead of being harsh on yourself, focus on getting back on track.

Keep in mind that consistency is crucial, not perfection.

# Challenge Your Sleep Sabotage

When you find yourself struggling to sleep, consider reframing your perspective. Instead of categorizing these nights as either fantastic or terrible, show yourself some kindness and acknowledge that not every night will be perfect. Remember, it's entirely normal to have nights that are a bit rough. You're not alone in this!

Instead of feeling disheartened, consider what you can learn from these experiences.

What habits or routines might be impacting your sleep?

How can you use that knowledge to make positive changes to your sleep patterns?

# Your Sleepiness Meter

You've heard of melatonin, the sleep-promoting hormone, but did you know your body has another clever way of measuring sleepiness? It's called adenosine, and think of it as your sleepiness meter!

Understanding how it works can help you feel more in control of your energy levels and sleep.

## How Adenosine Works

Imagine your alertness level as a gauge. When you wake up, it's nearly empty. But as the day goes on, the gauge fills with adenosine. The fuller it gets, the sleepier you feel.

Here's how it plays out:

**Morning Boost:** Waking up means low adenosine and high energy. Tackle those more demanding tasks and get your workout in!

**Mid-Day Dip:** Don't fight the natural afternoon slump! Instead of endless coffee, drink water, try a short walk, some daylight, or even a micro-power nap to reset your gauge.

**Evening Wind-Down:** As bedtime approaches, adenosine levels naturally rise again. Listen to this signal and enjoy calming activities to prepare for sleep.

**Caffeine Considerations:** Caffeine blocks adenosine from doing its job, which is why it feels energized. But timing matters! Caffeine too close to bedtime can throw off your whole sleep cycle.

## Tune Into Your Gauge

Understanding adenosine gives you a powerful tool. Plan your day around your body's natural peaks and dips for optimal energy and more restful sleep.

Here's one more way to use your sleepiness meter to your advantage:

**Mindful Moments:** When you notice tiredness creeping in, take a few minutes for mindful breathing or gentle stretching to help lower those adenosine levels.

## The Power of Paying Attention

By becoming aware of your internal sleepiness meter, you can make choices that support your energy and rest.

Your body is always talking - now you know how to listen!

Are you listening?

# Act on Your Sleep Knowledge

Inspired by Hannah, Sheila, and our other sleepy friends? Here's how to turn their experiences into your own sleep success story:

1   **Experiment:** Embrace your inner scientist! Channel Hannah and try limiting your time in bed. Or perhaps Sheila's unwavering evening unwind is more your style? Remember, sleep patterns are individual, and finding your sweet spot is crucial.

2   **Be a Detective:** What patterns do you see in your responses? This is your roadmap to unlocking better sleep. Are there specific triggers or habits that pop up? Identifying these will laser-focus your efforts.

3   **Choose One Change:** Sustainable sleep success isn't a sprint; it's a marathon. Focus on one achievable change: saying "no" to late-night snacks, creating a relaxing bedtime ritual, or establishing a consistent sleep schedule.

4   **The Power of Progress:** Acknowledge the changes you're already making, no matter how small! Your path to better sleep begins with courage – each step brings you closer.

5   **Identifying Potential Obstacles:** What might be keeping you from sleep success? Be ruthlessly honest with yourself! Is stress calling the shots? Is social media stealing your sleep? Recognizing these obstacles and a plan to navigate empowers you to overcome them.

## Unlocking Sleep Mastery

You're already taking the first crucial step toward better sleep. This isn't just about tips and tricks; it's about unlocking a new level of sleep mastery.

Imagine a sleep strategy so perfectly you, so filled with joy and wonder, that it feels almost magical. What if the key to those elusive, restful nights lies in a playful evening unwind, a quest to uncover the secrets of your sleep patterns, or a beautiful, calming ritual that speaks to your soul?

## Your Sleep Transformation Begins Tonight.

How can you make tonight the night? Imagine the extraordinary power you hold within—the power to close that frustrating sleep gap and unleash a ripple effect of well-being. Picture yourself approaching sleep with a sense of childlike wonder. What if a simple shift in perspective could unlock a wellspring of energy, creativity, and resilience?

## Embracing the Journey

Remember, even the most rewarding journeys have twists and turns. There will be nights of triumph and moments where you adjust your course. That's where the true magic of transformation unfolds.

# A Sleep Journey Continues

Once upon a time, there was Jessica, a busy mom who struggled with sleep. While she discovered some practical and effective tactics to improve her sleep, she realized she needed to continue building a lasting friendship with sleep. Would you like to revisit some tools and techniques that helped Jessica get back on track?

## Small Changes, Big Impact

Jessica knows that one bad night doesn't derail her progress. She focuses on what she can control, like gradually pushing her bedtime earlier to get those precious extra minutes of rest.

Instead of feeling defeated by the occasional setback, she focuses on the positive effects of consistent effort.

## Calm Your Mind

When racing thoughts strike, Jessica doesn't panic. She uses simple techniques, like a "brain dump" before bed or focusing on her breath, to gently redirect her mind toward calm.

Jessica understands that even small victories over mental distractions have a ripple effect on her sleep quality.

# Tracking Your Progress

Jessica discovered the advantages of tracking her sleep. Consistent wake-ups after a good night's sleep helped her feel refreshed, even after a rough night.

By tracking her sleep patterns, Jessica could celebrate her progress and focus on positive changes, no matter how small.

Jessica learned that she didn't have to change her lifestyle drastically to achieve the deep, rejuvenating sleep she deserved.

Suppose you're looking to improve your sleep quality. In that case, you can follow Jessica's lead and start tracking your sleep tonight to experience the difference it can make!

| Bedtime | Wake-up time | How did I feel? | Notes* |
|---------|--------------|-----------------|--------|
|         |              |                 |        |
|         |              |                 |        |
|         |              |                 |        |

\* Notes: Use this space to record any additional observations or factors that might have affected your sleep, both positively and negatively..

# Master Your Sleep Basics

Building better sleep habits is like constructing a well-crafted house—it takes the right tools for the job. This book offers tools for unlocking the potential already within you, with simple techniques to tap into your strengths and ways to leverage your determination for positive change.

## Crafting Your Building Blocks

### Self-Belief:
It starts with believing that improvement is possible. Practice replacing "I'm a bad sleeper" with "I'm capable of learning healthier sleep habits."
Just like a builder wouldn't start a project believing it's doomed to fail, start your sleep journey confidently in your ability to grow.

### The Sleep Detective:
Instead of fighting your sleep patterns, consider becoming an observer. A simple sleep log could provide valuable insights into what helps and hinders your rest. Understanding your ideal sleep conditions is critical – like piecing together clues to unlock a sleep mystery!

# Integrate Everyday Essentials

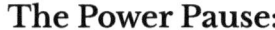

**The Power Pause:**
When worries or racing thoughts try to hijack your calm, stop the struggle. Take a slow, deep breath and return your focus to the present moment. For example, notice the feeling of your bedsheets against your skin or the sound of your own breathing.

**The "Park It" Pad:**
If your mind races at bedtime, keeping a notepad by your bed is helpful. Jotting down any nagging thoughts and reminding yourself, "I can address this tomorrow," can ease mental clutter. Just like jotting down a grocery list item helps clear it from your mind, this simple act can lessen mental clutter.

**Consistency over Perfection:**
Aiming to change everything overnight can lead to frustration. Start with a few adjustments you can realistically stick with. Imagine adding a new, sturdy beam to your "sleep house" each week—it creates a strong foundation over time.

# Activate Your Relaxation Response

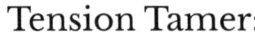

Tension Tamer:
Simple body scan meditation is a powerful tool that doesn't require external guidance. Start by lying comfortably and focusing on your breath for a few minutes. Then, slowly shift your attention to each body part (toes, feet, legs, etc.), noticing any sensations and consciously relaxing those muscles as you go.

**Reframing Restlessness:**
Instead of battling middle-of-the-night awakenings, try a counterintuitive approach. Gentle stretches, a calming podcast, or simply focusing on your breath can make rest productive even if sleep doesn't immediately return. Consider it a mini-break during construction – you're still progressing, even if it's not the main task.

**Bedroom Environment Audit:**
Even minor light, temperature, or noise adjustments can significantly impact sleep quality. Creating a cozy sleep sanctuary doesn't require a significant overhaul. Simple adjustments like blackout curtains or a thermostat tweak can create a cozy sleep sanctuary.

# Cultivate Your Resilience

**Experimentation is Key:**
What works wonders for one person might not be your ideal solution. Play around with the timing and application of these tools to find your perfect fit. The best builders try different materials and techniques to find what works!

**Kindness is Your Compass:**
Some nights will be harder than others. Instead of self-criticism, practice self-compassion and acknowledge your efforts. Remember, even experienced builders have setbacks—the key is to learn from them and keep going.

**Celebrate Progress:** Did you read for 15 minutes instead of scrolling before bed? That demonstrates self-control and intentionality—important strengths in crafting healthier habits! Did you manage to fall asleep after waking up?

Your balanced determination and willingness to try new techniques are making a difference!
Every step forward, no matter how small, is a testament to your commitment to improving your sleep.

Take a moment to reflect.

What new insights have you gained about your
sleep patterns and the power hidden within your habits?

What is a lingering question you still want to unravel,
or perhaps a surprising strength you've uncovered?

Start doing:

This journey is far from over. Think of the tools you've gathered as the start of something much bigger– a lifelong exploration of leveraging your immense capacity to create the deep, restorative rest that fuels your dreams.

Believe in your resilience,
dedication to well-being,
and ability to shape the sleep
that supports your best life.

Remember that your choices,
big and small, have the potential to
transform your sleep, one night at a time.

With every sunrise,
you can build upon what you've learned,
tweak those tools, and discover
even more effective ways to make sleep
your ally in living a vibrant, fulfilling life.

# Sleep and Me

As I closed my journal, a conversation unfolded between Sleep and Me...

*Dear Sleep,*

*Look at us now! I used to dread you, but now...it feels like we're a team.*
*Thank you for not giving up on me, even when I made it difficult.*
*This journey isn't over, but knowing you're*
*by my side makes all the difference.*

*Warmly, Me*

*Dearest Me,*

*You're right; we've come a long way! I'm proud of the effort you've put in.*
*Remember, our sleep relationship won't always be perfect.*
*Some nights will be easier than others.*
*But as long as we communicate and work together,*
*we'll return to those restful nights.*

*Sweet Dreams,*
*Sleep*

*Dear Sleep,*

*Thanks for reminding me that sleep is about progress, not perfection.*
*I'm finally starting to feel hopeful about this whole sleep thing.*
*And hey, it feels pretty good to have you on my team!*

*Rest well, Me.*

*My Dearest Me,*

*Get used to that hopeful feeling – it's a sign you're on the right track.*
*And remember, I'll always be here, ready to guide you*
*towards brighter tomorrows.*

*Rest well,*
*Sleep*

# The Sleep-Aligned Plan

*A framework to help you cultivate your
sleep friendship for restful nights*

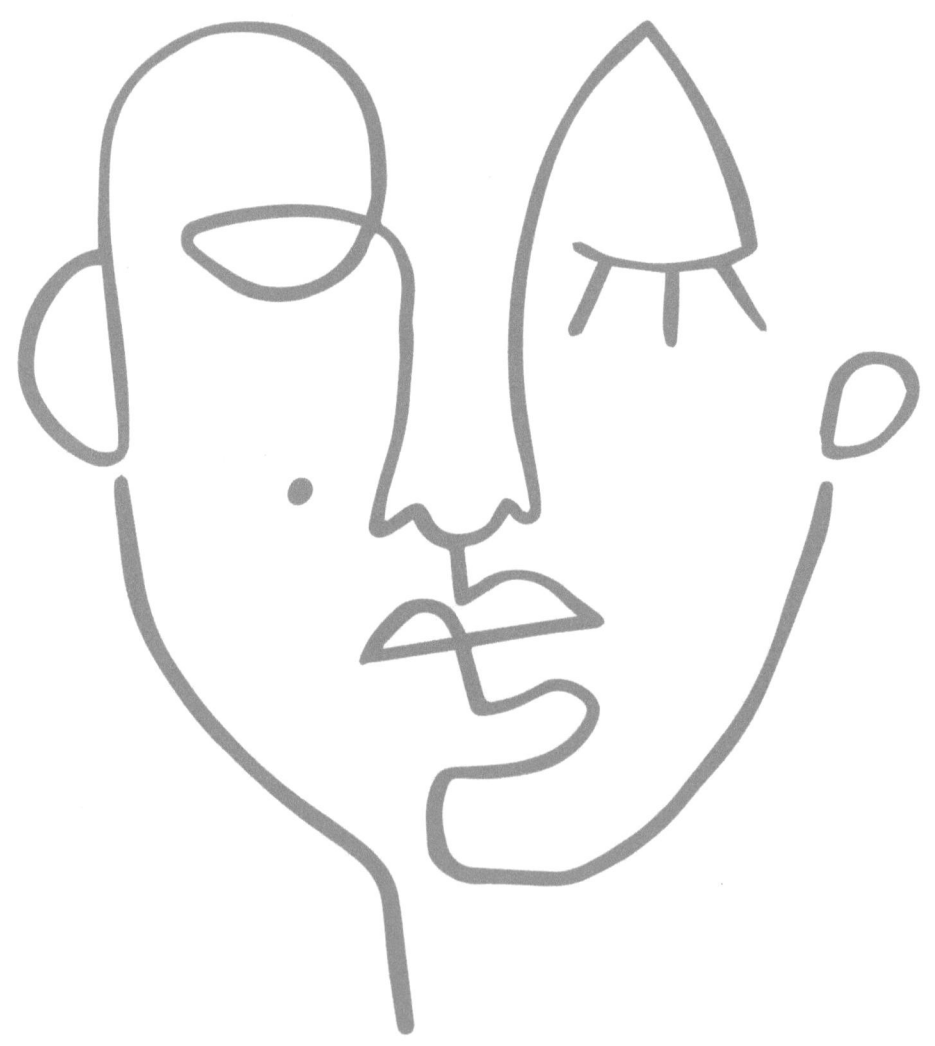

# The Sleep Aligned Plan

**A - Assess Your Sleep Story- Your Sleep "Why"**
What one change are you ready to make to improve your sleep quality, and why is this change necessary?

**L - Leverage Your Strengths - Your Sleep Strengths**
What strengths have helped you achieve quality sleep in the past, and how can you leverage them to continue improving your sleep routine?

**I - Ignite Your Sleep Spark - Does Your Plan Feel Right?**
How can you align your sleep goals and actions with your "why" and strengths to make sleep an exciting and joyful part of your life rather than a chore?

**G - Goal Setting for Sleep Success - Goals That Fit Your Life**
What specific actions can you take to ensure that your sleep goals align with your bigger picture and spark excitement and possibility?

## N - Navigate the Sleep Journey - Befriending the Challenges

What specific challenges do you anticipate while navigating your sleep journey, and how do you plan to overcome them?

## E - Emphasize the Power of Progress - Habits for Healthy Sleep

What two to three habits will you create to support your sleep goals? How can you ensure that your habits for better sleep align with your strengths and capacities?

## D - Develop Your Sleep Leadership - Weekly Sleep Check-Ins

To improve your sleep patterns, schedule a sleep check-in each week. During this time, reflect on your progress and identify how your unique abilities can help you sleep better.

Consider applying the skill stacking approach to determine which skills can improve your sleep. Some examples of skills that can be helpful for better sleep include exposure to daylight, relaxation techniques, meditation, and creating a comfortable sleep environment.

It's important to remember that some nights will be better than others. Therefore, it's essential to adapt your plan with kindness and allow yourself to adjust it as needed.

# The Sleep Alchemist

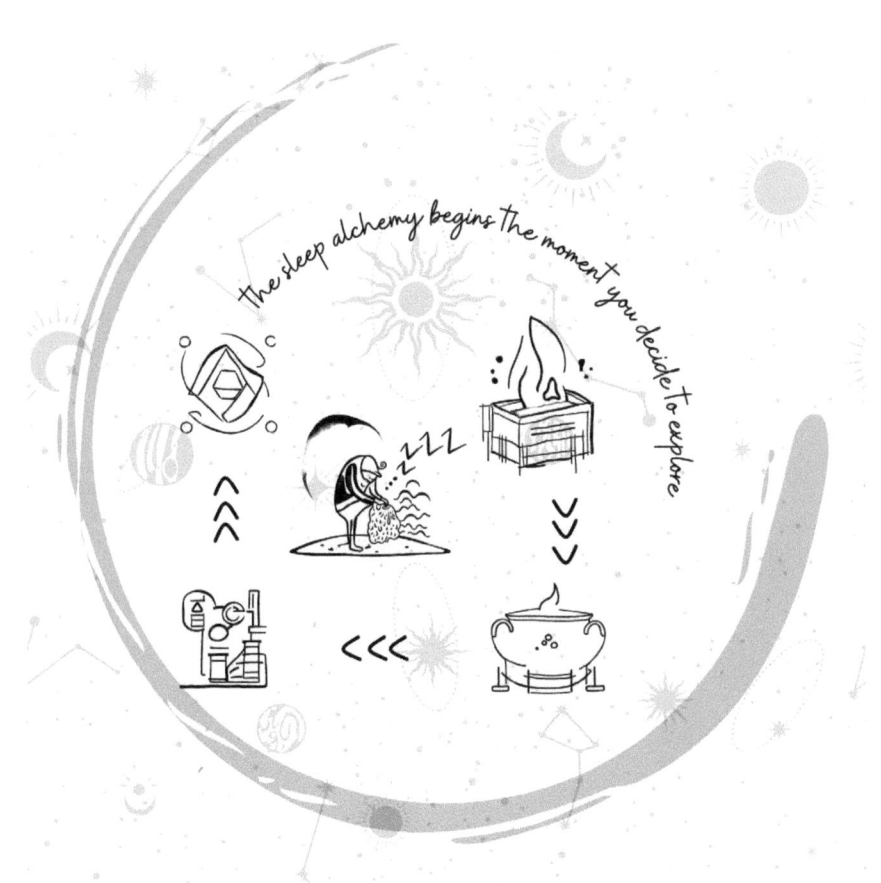

the sleep alchemy begins the moment you decide to explore

# Sleep Alchemy

*The art of alchemy has been known to offer transformative powers,
and this chapter draws inspiration from it to provide effective and practical
strategies and mindset shifts for improving sleep.*

*Like the ancient alchemists who strived to turn ordinary metals into gold, the
journey to peaceful sleep can be equally complicated and messy.*

*However, creativity, curiosity, and persistence can help you make significant
progress and gain invaluable insights.*

*So, let's play, embrace the transformative power of alchemy,
and take steps toward a better and more peaceful sleep.*

*- Bibi -*

*Please note that I use the term "Sleep Alchemist" and "Sleep Alchemy" is purely for
creative purposes and is fictitious. It does not represent any actual profession or medical
practice and should not be relied upon as such.*

# Awaken the Golden Potential
# Within Your Nights

The pillow's softness finally feels like an invitation, not a taunt. Your breath deepens, a gentle rhythm replacing the frantic pulse of worry. While the night might not always be perfect, there's a new-found sense of ease, a trust that your body remembers the way to rest. Days unfold with less fog, small moments of focus, and joy reemerging... and this is how it happened.

This change didn't happen overnight, nor was it about forcing yourself into a rigid mold. Instead, it began with awakening a hidden power within you. You began to understand the hidden language of your sleepless nights. You learned to work with, not against, your body and mind, gradually unearthing the restorative power hidden within.

The world knows of alchemists who sought to turn lead into gold, masters of fire and transformation. Yet, within you resides a different kind of alchemist—a Sleep Alchemist. Your workshop is the quiet of the night, and your vessel is not metal but your own weary body and restless mind. The 'base metal' you work with is the ache of exhaustion, the scattered fragments of anxious thoughts, and the heavy weight of frustration.

Yet, unlike the feeling of being trapped in a battle with your own body, the alchemist sees even the unrefined as brimming with potential. As the alchemist sees potential within the unrefined, so can you find the seeds of transformation within your sleeplessness.

Your fire is the gentle flame of self-awareness; your tools are the practices and insights you'll gather. You learn to observe how tiredness manifests, not as an enemy, but as a raw element to be understood. You experiment, discovering rituals that transmute worry into soothing rhythms and thoughts that splinter rest into a soft hum of acceptance.

The 'gold' a Sleep Alchemist seeks isn't the absence of all restless nights but something far more precious. It's the deep knowing that even within struggle, rest is possible. It's the rediscovery of your body's innate ability to heal. It's the newfound power to shape your relationship with sleep, not as a victim but as a co-creator of a more harmonious dance between waking and rest.

The path of a Sleep Alchemist isn't about following a rigid script but reclaiming your innate wisdom. It's about unearthing your hidden power to reshape your relationship with sleep, finding strength where you may only feel struggle.

The tools of this transformation lie within reach—in the gentle observation of your body's signals, experimentation with soothing practices, and the gradual shift from fighting sleeplessness to befriending it.

This journey is uniquely yours, woven with the threads of resilience, the ability to bend without breaking, and a spark of hope that whispers of untapped resources within. Becoming a Sleep Alchemist is a journey that anyone can embark on.

The Sleep Alchemy begins the moment you decide to explore

# What if exhaustion isn't your enemy but the raw material for the Sleep Alchemist's work?

Imagine your exhaustion not as a force that crushes you but as a dense, tangled mass of energy waiting to be shaped.

The Sleep Alchemist within you sees potential where you might only feel struggle. This alchemist gathers raw exhaustion, not to erase it, but to understand its texture.

Is the weariness a dull muscle ache, a relentless buzzing in your mind, or a sense of heaviness that defies reason?

Much like the alchemist observes the base metal, you begin your transformative work by observing your exhaustion with curiosity rather than fear.

The alchemist learns to soften that energy with the steady flame of conscious breathing, to guide it with gentle movements that release tension, and to quiet the mind's chatter, filtering out restless thoughts like impurities, allowing a state of calm to precipitate.

This shift in perspective is the foundation of the Sleep Alchemist's practice.

# The Exhaustion Ritual

This exercise can turn your exhausting experience into a moment of power. You can become a Sleep Alchemist, utilizing your internal state as a resource.

Your goal is to transform the negative perception of exhaustion into a creative force, which can be a powerful tool in facilitating better sleep.

Rather than viewing exhaustion as a burden, reframing it as a natural part of the creative process can help you harness its energy and channel it towards restful sleep.

By recognizing the value of exhaustion and using it to fuel your creativity, you can achieve a more positive outlook on your body's signals and enjoy a more restful and rejuvenating sleep experience.

It's mesmerizing how changing negative thought patterns can significantly impact your well-being. A shift in mindset can do wonders, especially regarding exhaustion and its effects on sleep. Rather than succumbing to feelings of overwhelm by exhaustion, shifting our perspective might involve finding ways to address and manage it, ultimately leading to better sleep.

And that's precisely what The Sleep Alchemist approach is about—it takes this idea to the next level by incorporating a ritualistic and empowering element, making the experience even more impactful and transformative for you.

# The Ritual

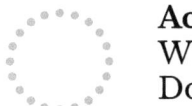

**Acknowledgement:**
When you feel exhausted in the evening, find a quiet place. Don't fight the feeling; welcome it consciously. "I am a Sleep Alchemist; this is my raw material."

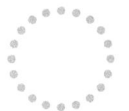

**Observation:**
Pay close attention to how exhaustion manifests in your body and mind. Describe its qualities in detail: Is it sharp and buzzing? Heavy and dragging? Use sensory language.

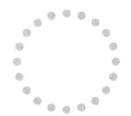

**Transmutation:**
Imagine your breath as a bellows, gently fanning a flame beneath your exhaustion. Visualize it softening, shifting, and becoming more malleable. Now, let this transformed energy move slowly through your body, finding areas of tension to soothe.

**Creation:**
Choose a simple, calming action fueled by your transformed exhaustion: slow stretches, sipping a warm beverage, or reading a calming book.

As a Sleep Alchemist, you hold the key to transforming exhaustion into a creative force that propels you towards a journey of restful sleep. You have the power to shape your sleep quality.

By keenly observing your body's signals and courageously experimenting with soothing practices, you can discover your inner strength and reshape your relationship with sleep.

It's crucial to attune to your natural rhythms and actively seek out activities that foster relaxation and peace.

So, embrace your inner Sleep Alchemist by incorporating calming rituals into your pre-sleep routine to signal to your body that it's time to wind down. And awaken the golden potential within your nights.

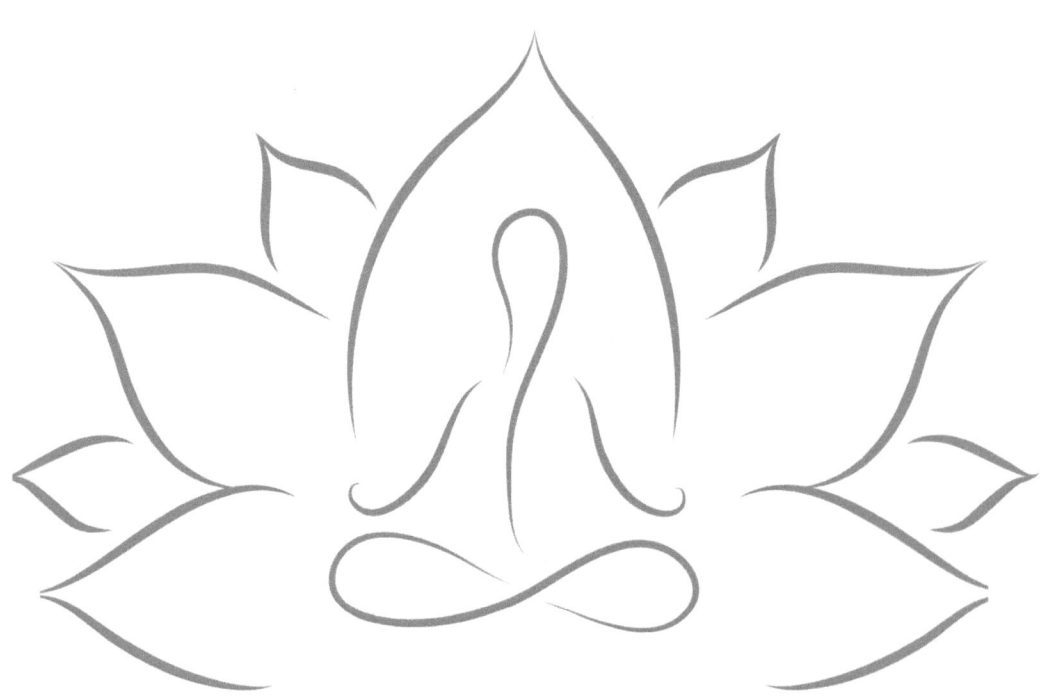

# Dreamcatcher Journaling

The Dreamcatcher Journaling exercise can help you connect your conscious mind with the unconscious, encouraging a sense of hopeful expectation around sleep.

By harnessing the subconscious power of sleep, you can improve your overall well-being, sleep quality, creativity, and happiness.

By filtering out worries and cultivating a mindset of possibility during your sleep, you can wake up feeling refreshed, motivated, and ready to tackle whatever challenges come your way.

The Sleep Alchemist approach is a potent technique that merges imagery and journaling. This method helps you connect with your intuitive and creative side, allowing you to access your innermost thoughts and feelings about sleep. Doing so can overcome mental barriers preventing you from getting the rest you need for a healthy mind and body.

What if your relationship with sleep
could be shaped and transformed,
not by external forces,
but by your own innate wisdom?

# The Practice

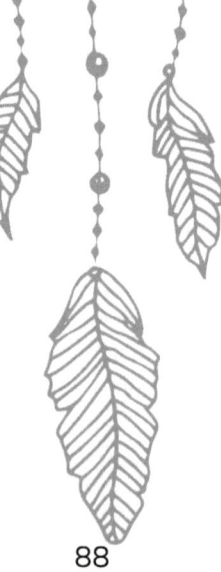

**The Dreamcatcher:** Begin by drawing a simple dreamcatcher. This represents your mind's ability to filter and transform worries.

**The Web:** Let your worries spill onto the paper around the dreamcatcher. They can be as messy, tangled, and illogical as you need them to be.

**Transformation:** Now, imagine each worry caught in the dreamcatcher's web. Visualize it shrinking, softening, or changing into something less threatening

**Possibility Seeds:** Around the edge of your dreamcatcher, write down a few small hopes, dreams, or simple pleasures you are open to experiencing in your sleep or the following day.

# The Alchemical Cycle of Slumber

Welcome to a transformative journey that can significantly enhance your sleep quality and overall well-being. In this chapter, you will discover the tools and knowledge to turn your sleep struggles into restorative rest and lead a more fulfilling life.

As you delve deeper into the exercises, you can uncover the secrets of being a Sleep Alchemist. You can learn how to use your transformative power to turn the base metal of sleep struggles into the gold of deep, restorative rest.

To guide this transformation, let's explore the power of rituals. Rituals can be powerful tools for creating and reinforcing habits. They can have a deeper meaning, making them more potent than mere routines. By adding a sense of importance or ceremony to a task, a ritual can help create a stronger emotional connection to the activity, making it more likely that you will continue to perform it over time.

Utilizing the Alchemical Cycle of Slumber as your guide, you can approach your sleep issues fresh. This playful approach can help you create new, healthier habits.

Remember that you are not just a participant but the master of your sleep transformation. With every step you take, you can be one step closer to achieving the restful sleep you hope for. Take your time, explore every facet of the Alchemical Cycle of Slumber, and let the power of transformation guide you towards a better, more restful life.

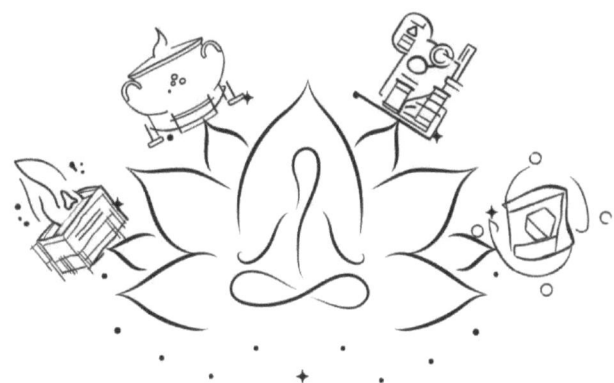

# 1. Calcination: Unveiling the Impurities of Sleep

**The Alchemist's Work:**
In this initial stage, calcination, the alchemist breaks down the raw metal with fire, separating impurities and creating a foundation for change.

**The Sleep Alchemist:**
Just as the alchemist separates impurities and creates a foundation for change through calcination, The Sleep Alchemist creates a solid foundation for transformation by breaking down the barriers that prevent healthy sleep patterns.

## 1.1 Transmuting Sleep Struggles into Spells of Empowerment

Just like how the alchemist breaks down raw metal with fire to create gold, you can transform your sleep struggles into something valuable by understanding the Language of Sleep.

By learning to speak, think, feel, and act about your sleep in a way that empowers you, you can turn your sleep struggles into a foundation for change.

Your sleep struggles can be the impurities that must be identified and separated. But remember, they can also be transformed into something precious with the right mindset and approach. This is not just a challenge; it's an opportunity for positive change that can transform your sleep and life.

Remember, just like how the alchemist creates gold from metal, you can create better sleep from your struggles by understanding the language of sleep and using the knowledge to intentionally build a strong foundation for transformation.

**Worksheet:**

To improve the quality of your sleep, it's essential to pay attention to how you talk about it. List the negative words and phrases you currently use to describe your sleep, such as 'I always wake up tired' or 'I can never fall asleep quickly.'

Let's turn these negative self-talk into potions of power! Instead of 'I always wake up tired,' you could try, 'My body is learning to rest deeply,' or 'With each night, I grow closer to the refreshing sleep I deserve.'

Use this to craft a new sleep language that replaces the negativity and frustration with your desired optimistic words or images.

Doing so allows you to set yourself up for a more restful and rejuvenating night's sleep.

| Negative self-talk | Replace with optimistic words |
|---|---|
|  |  |
|  |  |
|  |  |
|  |  |

## 1.2 The Crucible of Sleep: Separating Obstacles from Essence

This step involves identifying and understanding the root causes of your sleep struggles, both internal and external.

### Worksheet:

To address your struggles with falling asleep, you can create a simple, three-column chart.

Label the first column as "Struggle" and identify the particular challenge preventing you from getting restful sleep. For example, you might write, "I can't fall asleep."

In the second column, distinguish between internal and external factors contributing to sleep difficulty.

For instance, if your mind is racing with thoughts, label the factor "internal."

In contrast, a noisy neighbor would be labeled "external." Finally, in the third column, brainstorm one small change that you can potentially make to address the issue.

Using this worksheet, you'll be able to identify your specific sleep struggles and take actionable steps toward finding a solution.

| Struggle | Internal or external | One small change |
|----------|---------------------|------------------|
|          |                     |                  |
|          |                     |                  |

## 1.3 Consecrating the Grimoire of Sleep

This is a crucial step, where you create a guidebook to address your sleep struggles and the outcomes you want. This guidebook can become your sacred 'chamber of transformation.'

Understanding that the road to better sleep is not a straight path is helpful. It's a cyclical journey that involves learning, adapting, growing, and refining. It can be challenging sometimes, but embracing your progress, celebrating your achievements, and staying hopeful for the future is equally important.

By tracking your experiences and insights in a dedicated sleep guidebook, you can better understand your relationship with sleep and find ways to improve it.

**Worksheet:**

To enhance the effectiveness of your sleep guide, start by creating an "Emblem of Transformation" on the first page and make it your Grimoire of Sleep. This emblem can be a simple droodle representing the sleep relationship you want.

By consecrating your Grimoire of Sleep in this way, you can better connect with your sleep goals and intentions, resulting in a more effective and fulfilling experience. [see page 127)

# 2. Dissolution: Crafting Elixirs of Rest

**The Alchemist's Work:**
The alchemist dissolves the raw materials in a liquid medium, promoting a state of receptive change.

**The Sleep Alchemist:**
Just as the alchemist dissolves raw materials in a liquid medium to promote change, the Sleep Alchemist introduces practices to balance and dissolve the "impurities" of sleeplessness. Processes involve change, in which the original substance is transformed into something new and improved.

## 2.1 Alchemy of the Mundane:

Did you know that sometimes, the most mundane activities can become powerful rituals if you approach them with intention and care?

Take, for instance, preparing yourself for a good night's sleep. A few simple steps can transform this into a soothing and calming experience.

Start by brewing yourself a sleep preparation elixir made from carefully chosen tea to help relax your mind and body.

Then, dim the lights to create a peaceful and restful atmosphere, perfect for a more restorative sleep.

Lastly, change into comfortable loungewear to signal to your body and mind that it's time to unwind and relax.

By approaching these simple acts with mindfulness and intention, you can transform them into potent rituals supporting your physical, mental, and emotional well-being and ultimately improve your sleep quality.

## 2.2 Crafting the Spell of Harmonious Days

With a packed schedule, it can be easy to habitually reduce sleep to meet deadlines. But know that your daily schedule significantly impacts your sleep quality? Instead of treating sleep as an afterthought, let's craft harmonious days and elixirs of rest that support restful nights.

One way to achieve this is by mapping your ideal energy flow. Visualize your energy levels throughout the day following a wave pattern with highs and lows. You can create your ideal flow by noting when you naturally feel energized, focused, or need a quiet recharge.

It's also crucial to consider sleep a sacred time. Protect your sleep time fiercely once you've identified your natural energy peaks and dips. Think of it as your "Sleep Incubation Period"—the time that nourishes your inner Sleep Alchemist.

However, it's important to remember that schedules are helpful tools, not unbreakable rules. Listen to your body and be flexible on days that don't go as planned.

Try the Energy Awareness exercise to start your journey towards a better sleep schedule. With each step, you'll be closer to crafting a harmonious spell of restful days and peaceful nights.

## Energy Awareness Worksheet

For a few days, pay close attention to your energy patterns. Here's how to get started:

**Energy Mapping:** Notice when you experience energy peaks, steady flow, and the need to recharge.

**Identifying Friction:** Where do your energy cycles clash with your current schedule. List at least three areas.

**Your Harmony Spell:** For each area of friction, consider the following:

How can you shift the timing of the activity for better alignment?

How can you add a quick ritual (movement break, meditation, calming tea) to counteract the negative effects?

**Choose Your Path:** Pick one adjustment and consciously implement it. Celebrate every step you take toward creating an elixir of rest that aligns with your needs.

| Time of the day | Energy level (high, medium, low) | Activities | Notes (emotions, thoughs, stress level) |
| --- | --- | --- | --- |
| | | | |
| | | | |
| | | | |
| | | | |
| | | | |

Identifying Friction:

Your Harmony Spell

Area of Friction:

Shifting Timing:

Quick Ritual:

Choose Your Path

I will implement the following adjustment:

I will celebrate my progress by:

## 2.3 The Alchemical Chart of Inner Strengths

If you're looking for a personalized plan to improve your sleep, nothing beats leveraging your strengths, the core of who you are. You can create a personalized plan to improve your sleep by tapping into your unique strengths.

The key is to truly understand your strengths and find ways to connect them to restful practices. This may require deep reflection and brainstorming, but the results will be well worth it.

Identify your top 3 character strengths, including things you enjoy doing. (You can take a free VIA Character Strengths assessment on VIACharacter.org.) By identifying your top three character strengths, you can gain insights into what drives you, what you enjoy doing, and where you can excel.

Prepare a sheet in your sleep guide with three columns: one for your strength, one for brainstorming how it could help improve your sleep, and one for actionable ideas (think rituals).

Fill out the columns and take some time to reflect on which connection between your strengths and sleep surprised you the most and which idea feels the most exciting or empowering to try.

Encouraging playfulness and exploration over rigid "right" answers is essential. Hopefully, this exercise will spark new ideas for personalized and meaningful rituals to improve sleep.

So go ahead, try it, and experience the difference it makes in your life!

# 3. Separation: Distilling Resilience from Setbacks

**The Alchemist's Work:**
With careful manipulation, the alchemist separates the refined elements from the remaining waste.

**The Sleep Alchemist:**
Like an alchemist, takes the raw materials of their sleep habits and refines them into a more restful and rejuvenating experience. With perseverance and commitment, the Sleep Alchemist separates the refined elements of healthy sleep from the remaining waste of bad habits, just as an alchemist separates valuable metals from dross.

## 3.1 Transmutin Anxious Thoughts with the Elixir of Perspective

If you're struggling with anxious thoughts and restlessness, remember that achieving perfect sleep won't happen overnight. Instead of viewing setbacks as failures, consider them experiments and take note of your triggers and resilience to learn from them.

To alleviate tension, you can try practicing **thought alchemy**. This technique involves transforming your worries into neutral thoughts. Choose a common worry and create a simple symbol that represents it. When the uneasiness comes to mind, visualize the symbol disintegrating slowly and being replaced by a neutral image. This visual exercise can help you shift your focus away from negative thoughts and reduce anxiety.

Another technique is **thought restructuring**, replacing negative sleep thoughts with more compassion. Instead of telling yourself, "I'm too worried to sleep," try saying, "It's okay to be worried, but I can still rest and relax. I'll deal with my worries in the morning when I feel refreshed."

Finally, **Stimulus control** is a potent sleep alchemy that can help transform your sleep struggles into gold. Training your brain to associate your bed and bedroom with relaxation and sleep can create a magical sleep environment that promotes restfulness and rejuvenation.

To practice this stimulus control, it's best to deliberately separate from devices and stimulating activities before bed. This means you avoid using electronic devices such as your phone, tablet, or laptop or engaging in activities requiring mental or physical stimulation.

## 3.2 Concocting the Brew of Resilience

Embrace the art of Concocting the Brew of Resilience to transform challenging nights into opportunities for growth. Rather than dwelling on imperfections, celebrate the small victories—those moments when you made a conscious choice to support your well-being.

Perhaps you resisted the urge to check your phone, practiced deep breathing exercises, or acknowledged your struggles with kindness. Every act of self-compassion, no matter how small, is an ingredient in this potent brew.

Jot down these victories in your sleep guidebook, reminding you of your resilience. As your "Brew of Resilience" grows more robust, so will your ability to navigate sleepless nights with grace and self-assurance.

Remember, resilience extends beyond sleep. Celebrating wins like asking for help, setting boundaries, or taking a break when needed are all essential components of your overall well-being, fueling your capacity for restful sleep.

# 4. Conjunction: Forging the Golden Sleep

**The Alchemist's Work:**
The alchemist recombinates the purified elements, forging a new, higher-quality creation.

**The Sleep Alchemist:**
Just as the alchemist takes purified elements and forges them into a higher-quality creation, the Sleep Alchemist creates a new level of mastery by combining different techniques and practices to create a more restful and rejuvenating sleep experience.

Both the Alchemist and the Sleep Alchemist seek to transform and improve upon what already exists, creating something new and better.

## 4.1 The Ever-Unfolding Grimoire of Sleep

The Ever-Unfolding Grimoire of Sleep is invaluable for anyone who values restful nights. You can pinpoint what works best for you by tracking your sleep patterns and successes. This helps you improve the quality of your sleep and gives you a sense of control over your sleep habits.

The empowerment of taking charge of your sleep can be deeply healing. Decorating your sleep guide with small drawings, symbols representing emotions, and stickers can make it a treasure trove of insights and self-reflection.

So start keeping a sleep guide today and let it guide you towards more restful nights and happier mornings!

## 4.2 Refining the Sleep Alchemist's Potion

Here's the thing: perfecting your sleep potion is ongoing. As your body and mind evolve, so should your sleep rituals and elixirs.

Don't settle for a one-size-fits-all approach to sleep. Instead, take an active role in refining your sleep potion based on your unique needs and preferences.

Maybe you've discovered that moving your body earlier in the day helps you feel more relaxed come bedtime. Another tip is to stay hydrated by drinking plenty of water in the afternoon. And don't underestimate the power of positive self-talk - it can go a long way in promoting healthy sleep habits, including gratitude practices.

Bettering your sleep potion is an active process, not a passive one. Take the time to listen to your body and experiment with different sleep rituals and elixirs. You might just find the perfect formula for a blissful night's rest.

## 4.3 Recognizing Moments of Deep Rest

Paying attention to moments of deep rest is essential to forging the golden sleep. These moments can be elusive; therefore, take a moment to listen to your body. Once you've identified these moments, recreate them as often as possible.

### Restful Sleep
- When do you typically sleep well?
- Do you have difficulty falling asleep or staying asleep?
- What are the common factors that contribute to your restful sleep?
- How do you typically feel the next day after a peaceful night?

### Positive Triggers
- Name a few positive triggers that make it easier for you to relax and feel at ease?
- What steps can you take to optimize or maximize these triggers?

### Moments of Deep Rest
- When do you typically feel most rested and rejuvenated?
- What patterns or behaviors lead up to those moments of deep rest?

### Action Plan
- Based on your answers to the above questions, what steps can you take to prioritize your sleep and increase your moments of deep rest?What patterns or behaviors lead up to those moments of deep rest?
- What barriers might you face when incorporating them, and how can you overcome them?

## 4.4 Celebrate the Gold

Congratulations on your achievement as a Sleep Alchemist! By turning your sleep struggles into gold, you have stepped towards a healthier and happier life. It's crucial to continue acknowledging and utilizing your strengths to support healthy sleep habits.

Remember, quality sleep is essential for your well-being and the well-being of those around you. When you wake up feeling genuinely refreshed and energized, you can tackle the day with renewed vigor, and this positivity will radiate to your loved ones and colleagues. With the right tools and support, you can achieve the sleep you need to live your best life. So keep celebrating your successes and keep striving for better sleep!

**4.4 Planting the Seeds of Dream Wisdom** is an advanced, powerful, and effective technique for achieving calm and restful sleep.

By planting seeds of intention in your mind before going to bed, you can consciously direct the focus of your subconscious mind towards calming and peaceful dreams.

However, it is essential to note that the results of this technique may vary from person to person, and having vivid dreams is not necessarily the goal.

With regular practice, you can draw from your inner wisdom's vast potential and use the power of your dreams to achieve deep relaxation and personal growth.

Dream incubation can provide valuable insight and clarity, helping you transform your waking life and achieve balance, peace, and joy.

# The Ever-Evolving Sleep Alchemist

The path of the Sleep Alchemist is an ever-evolving cycle, much like the changing of the seasons. From adjusting sleep environments to implementing new positive triggers, the Sleep Alchemist's work is never finished.

Practising Sleep Alchemy is not about perfection; it's about learning to dance with the ebb and flow of restlessness, listening to your body's whispers, and cultivating a deep sense of trust in your innate wisdom.

With time and practice, you'll see the fruits of your labor -  gold - a newfound sense of ease, a more harmonious relationship with sleep, and a deeper connection to your inner alchemist and the world around you.

May this journey bring you peace, joy, and a sense of empowerment that stays with you
long after your head hits the pillow.

# Embracing Sleep:
# A Journey of Self-Care and Transformation

*Dear reader,*

*My hope is that these pages will be a trusted companion, a source of guidance and inspiration as you embark on your empowering journey to build that strong, optimistic relationship with sleep.*

*Remember, change takes time. Start with small victories, celebrate every slight improvement, and be kind to yourself on the more challenging nights. With each step, you'll discover more restful nights, brighter mornings, and the transformative power of sleep.*

*Don't be afraid to experiment with different sleep improvement techniques, such as establishing a consistent sleep schedule, creating a relaxing bedtime routine, or adjusting your sleep environment. Find what works best for you, and make sleep a joyful part of your self-care routine.*

*Imagine the endless possibilities that await when you're genuinely well-rested – it's not just a dream, it's a gift you deserve!*

*With warmth and support,*
*Bibi*

# APPENDIX

# The Power of Personalized Solutions!

While we all experience sleep differently, certain struggles tend to crop up for many of us. As your knowledge of sleep has grown, you've discovered that the most effective strategies are the ones tailored to your individual needs. The challenges we face, and the solutions most likely to work, often change with different stages of life.

The following appendix breaks down common sleep struggles, offering tailored tips and techniques to help you conquer the obstacles specific to your situation.

Think of it as your personalized guide to restful nights,
no matter where you are on life's journey.

# Internal Struggles
## Mental Overdrive

### The Overthinking Trap
When you experience racing thoughts as you try to fall asleep, it can feel like your mind is replaying the day's events or worrying about future scenarios, making it impossible to switch off. This happens because stress, perfectionism, or a tendency to dwell on details can keep your brain in overdrive long after the day is done.

**Turn it around:** Practice "thought stopping" to break the cycle. Use breathing exercises or audio tracks to redirect your focus.

### Existential Questions
When faced with big life questions, pondering one's purpose, worrying about the future, and concerns about the present, it can feel like one's mind is constantly racing. This is often due to significant life transitions, responsibilities, and a sense of "time running out" that can lead to worry and introspection. It's understandable to feel this way, especially during significant life changes and transitions.

**Turn it around:** Journal to capture insights, build a support system, and practice mindfulness to calm your mind.

## The "What If?" Spiral

Dwelling on worst-case scenarios and potential negative outcomes can make you feel anxious and unable to relax. This kind of overthinking usually happens when a situation is uncomfortable or uncertain. Uncertainty is a natural worry trigger, and focusing on the uncontrollable amplifies anxiety.

**Turn it around:** These thoughts can be pretty stressful, but remember challenging any "what if" thoughts that come to mind is important. Ask yourself if they are realistic or if they are catastrophic. Instead of worrying about things out of your control, focus on what you can do now. Consider the worst possible outcome, the best possible outcome, and what is most likely to happen. This will help you gain perspective and reduce anxiety.

## Chaotic Schedules

Maintaining a consistent sleep schedule on weekends can be challenging, and you may catch up on missed sleep for hours. Factors such as shared living spaces and different schedules can compound the chaos. While it is understandable to want to relax and enjoy the weekends, doing so can lead to a lack of routine and a disruption in your sleep patterns.

**Turn it around:** Aim for slightly earlier weekend wake-ups, communicate with roommates, and use earplugs or eye masks when needed.

## The Super Early Shift

If you tend to be an early bird, you may find that your sleep schedule feels out of sync with those around you. However, embracing an earlier schedule also offers you a unique opportunity to enjoy peaceful mornings and a different perspective on the day. It's natural to experience shifting sleep patterns; there's nothing wrong with preferring to wake up earlier. Feeling isolated and misaligned with others' schedules can sometimes creep in at night, making you restless.

**Turn It Around:** Own Your Early Hours: Use the extra time for activities you enjoy—meditation, reading, journaling, or a leisurely breakfast while everyone sleeps. Explore new hobbies, like birdwatching or early morning yoga, specifically suited for those tranquil morning hours. Don't force yourself to stay up late if it feels wrong.

# Emotional Turmoil

## Haunting Regrets

Past choices or missed opportunities sometimes resurface, making it challenging to fall asleep peacefully. This can be particularly common during certain life stages when we feel like time is running out, leading to self-criticism and dwelling on regrets. It's understandable to feel this way, but it's important to remember that dwelling on the past won't change it. Instead, focus on the present moment and what you can do to create a better future.

**Turn it around:** Remember, it's normal to look back. Let past experiences inspire what you do next. Acknowledge past regrets, but use them as fuel for positive growth. Ask, "What would I do differently now?"

## Dreams of Missed Opportunities

Vivid dreams about past mistakes, unmet potential, or paths not taken can leave you feeling regretful or frustrated upon waking, influencing your mood and disrupting sleep. Our dreams often reflect grief, anxieties, and deep-seated worries, and regret is a powerful emotion that can resurface in our subconscious while we sleep. These dreams can be your mind's way of processing unresolved feelings or highlighting areas where you might crave change in your current life.

**Turn it around:** Journaling about these dreams helps you understand your fears and regrets. Use those insights as fuel for growth and present-day action. Practice reframing negative self-talk with positive affirmations.

## The Empty Nest Blues

Experiencing sadness, loneliness, or a sense of lost purpose after children leave home can be challenging. This major life transition disrupts routines and changes family dynamics. It shifts feelings of identity, often leading to sleepless nights filled with worry or simply due to a quiet house. It's completely normal to feel this way, and it's important to remember that you're not alone.

**Turn it around:** Explore new hobbies and interests you didn't have time for. Focus on building connections outside of your immediate family circle.

# Seeking Control

## Revenge Bedtime Procrastination
Staying up late to reclaim personal time after a long day, even if you know it means being tired the next day - this feeling is quite common. It happens when you feel like work or responsibilities dominate your waking hours, leaving you with a desire for even a little bit of "me time."

**Turn it around:** Reframe your early mornings. Instead of seeing them as lost sleep, use them for enjoyable solo activities before the demands of the day set in. This can include reading a book, taking a relaxing walk, or enjoying a morning coffee or tea while getting to know the day.

## FOMO and Late Nights
It can be challenging to switch off and get a good night's sleep when you feel the need to constantly check your phone for notifications, social media, and news or stay on top of your never-ending to-do list. This can be incredibly challenging when you have a busy schedule, are pressured to excel in every aspect of your life, and fear missing out on important events or opportunities.

**Turn it around:** It's okay to take breaks and unplug - it's actually good for you! Make time for yourself, limit phone use, prioritize face-to-face interactions, reflect on accomplishments, and plan for the next day.

# Sleep Environment & Physical Factors

## External Disruptors

### The Noise Factor

Loud neighbors, traffic, and even a partner's breathing disrupt your sleep and leave you groggy in the morning. Unfortunately, this is a common problem for many people due to noise pollution being a part of many living situations. Sensitivity to sound also varies, making some people more prone to sleep disturbance.

**Turn it around:** White noise machines or earplugs can be surprisingly effective. Make the noise part of a meditation practice to change your perspective.

### The Nighttime Shuffle

Endless wake-ups with children – whether infants need feedings, toddlers with nightmares, or teens sneaking out – disrupt your sleep and lead to chronic exhaustion. This happens because parenting naturally comes with fragmented sleep, especially during certain stages of childhood

**Turn it around:** Create clear bedtime routines for children to encourage better sleep hygiene early. Team up with your partner, ask for help, and take strategic naps (where possible) to lessen the load.

# The Body's Needs

## The Temperature Tango

Feeling too hot (night sweats, stuffy rooms) or too cold (shivering, icy feet) can make it difficult to fall asleep or cause frequent wake-ups. The ideal sleep temperature is individual, and it's in a narrow range. Changes in body temperature regulation, room temperature, or even bedding choices can make all the difference in sleep quality. So, it's essential to maintain a comfortable sleep environment to ensure a good night's rest.

**Turn it around:**Create a well-tempered and ventilated sleeping environment. Invest in breathable sleepwear and, if necessary, explore cooling pillows and mattress pads.

## Sleep-Stealing Discomfort

Physical pain, aches, and an uncomfortable mattress or pillow can make falling or staying asleep difficult. When physical discomfort becomes a distraction, it can cause restlessness as you try to find a comfortable position. This restlessness can lead to fragmented sleep, making you tired and groggy the next day.

**Turn it around:** Assess your sleep setup. Is your mattress supportive? Does your pillow cause neck pain? Invest in ergonomic upgrades as needed. Stretching before bed can also be helpful.

# Disrupted Routines

## The Disappearing Sleep Anchor

Without the structure of a work schedule, your sleep-wake cycle feels adrift, leading to fragmented sleep. This happens because work often provides a sleep anchor, and its absence disrupts your body's natural cues. As a result, bedtime drifts later, making it challenging to maintain a healthy sleep routine.

**Turn it around:**Create a new routine with regular mealtimes and activities. If you don't need to be up, maintain a consistent wake-up and bedtime.

## Retirement = Restless

Without work's mental and physical stimulation, you may experience lingering unease, especially at night. Transitioning from stimulating work is a significant shift, and feeling a void is expected as one's identity and purpose change.

**Turn it around:** Rediscover hobbies, try new things, or volunteer. Physical activity is essential. This transition is a temporary adjustment period, and restful sleep will likely return.

# Relationship Dynamics

## Shared Space, Different Needs

### The Battle of the Bedroom

When your partner snores loudly, keeps you up all night, or tosses and turns restlessly, it can be frustrating and lead to resentment. These issues can arise from differences in lifestyle habits and evolving sleep patterns that cause misalignment between couples.

**Turn it around:** Sharing a bed can be lovely, but it's important to prioritize open communication and problem-solving when sleep needs differ. Addressing issues like snoring, experimenting with separate blankets, or adjusting bedtimes slightly to better align schedules can help. White noise may also be helpful for light sleepers.

### The Loneliness Challenge

A silent house can amplify feelings of isolation, making it challenging to feel calm at bedtime. Significant life changes can disrupt social circles, and humans thrive on connection. Sleep's absence can impact restless nights and a lack of rejuvenation in the morning.

**Turn it around:** Rekindle friendships, make new connections, and find community through hobbies or volunteering.

# Caring for Others

## The Emotions of Caregiving

Caring for a loved one can be emotionally and physically demanding, leaving you feeling worried and stressed. Whether it's an elderly parent, a child with special needs, or a sick partner, the weight of responsibility can keep your mind racing and disrupt your sleep. You may find yourself waking frequently to check on them or lying awake with anxiety, as the disrupted routines and emotional toll take a toll on your overall well-being.

**Turn it Around:** Build a support system for yourself—self-compassion and help from family and friends. Prioritize stress-reducing activities, even briefly, and practice mindfulness to calm your mind before bed. It is a privilege to have the capacity to care for a loved one, but you can still become tired - even exhausted.

## Caring for an Elderly Parent with Dementia

Watching a parent gradually lose their memory and cognitive abilities can be an incredibly emotional and challenging experience. The feelings of grief, sadness, and helplessness can feel overwhelming as you witness the person you once knew slip away. The constant demands of caregiving may disrupt your routines, leaving you exhausted and worried about their well-being and the challenges ahead.

**Turn it Around:**
Support groups designed for caregivers of individuals with dementia can provide valuable knowledge and assistance. Carve out time for self-care activities that bring you joy and relaxation, even if it's just for a few minutes each day. Taking care of yourself will enable you to provide better care for your parent.

# The Mind-Body Connection

## The Power of Dreams

### Vivid Nightmares

Disturbing and intense dreams, often referred to as nightmares, can leave you feeling shaken and anxious. These dreams can be so vivid and realistic that they may make it difficult to fall back asleep or even wake you up in distress. Recurring nightmares can be caused by several factors, including unresolved stress, trauma, and other underlying psychological factors.

**Turn it Around:** Changing the storyline of negative dreams can help reduce their impact on emotional well-being. To do this, you can try rewriting the script of the negative dream to change the outcome and make it less disturbing.

To interrupt and change the negative dream, try recalling it in detail and use your imagination to tweak the storyline unexpectedly. Think of yourself as an inner superhero who can alter the dream's course. After that, practice visualizing this new dream version in your mind's eye. Try to make the new script as vivid as possible. Repeat this process a few times over a few days or weeks.

With time and practice, this approach can help you desensitize to negative dreams and reduce their impact on your emotional well-being.

## Dreams Better Than Reality

Have you ever experienced a feeling where your dreams become so vivid and enjoyable that you resist waking up? The soft glow of your dream feels much more appealing than the harsh ring of an alarm clock. If yes, then you may have wondered why this happens. When real life feels stressful, unfulfilling, or overwhelming, dreams can offer an escape or an environment where you have more control. So, it's not uncommon to feel this way when going through a stressful phase in life.

**Turn it Around:** Examine your waking life – are there areas where you need more fulfilling experiences or greater autonomy? Mindfulness techniques can help you stay present when you wake up, easing the disappointment of leaving your dream world.

# Ambition's Impact

## Ambition on Overdrive

Equating long hours with success, seeing sleep as an obstacle, and feeling exhaustion like a badge of honor are some things that can happen when one has an intense drive to achieve and pressure to prove oneself.

**Turn it around:** Remember, sleep fuels goals. Track productive vs. busy hours. Create a post-work buffer zone.

## Sleep Envy & The "Shoulds"

Comparing yourself to others creates guilt about your struggles because constant online comparison is a trap. The curated moments we see on social media platforms don't reflect real life, and this can make us feel like everyone else is living a perfect life while we struggle to keep up.

**Turn it around:** Ditch comparison, focus on your journey, and celebrate small wins. Reflect on what you already have that you might wish for. The power of journaling as a solution might help reframe unhelpful comparisons

## The Wisdom of Worry

A lifetime of experiences can create a wellspring of wisdom as we age. Still, it can also lead to contemplating big questions or reflecting on past regrets at bedtime, making it difficult to find peace and drift off to sleep. This stage of life invites reflection and taking stock of our journey, making it all the more important to find meaning and purpose as the years pass.

**Turn It Around:** Journaling for Perspective: Use your journal to acknowledge worries and capture the valuable insights and hard-earned wisdom you've accumulated. Consider starting a 'gratitude list' to counterbalance anxieties with an appreciative lens.

# Technology's Influence

## The Revenge of the Screen

The blue light from screens suppresses melatonin, making it even harder to resist the "just one more episode" trap. You feel stuck, knowing that you should go to sleep but unable to tear yourself away from the screen. Screens are incredibly stimulating and addictive, and it's easy to lose track of time and stay up far later than you intended.

**Turn it around:** Strict "screens off" time at least an hour before bed. Use nighttime filters on devices. Replace late-night screen time with calming activities like reading or gentle stretches.

## The Phantom Buzz

The constant notifications and the fear of missing out (FOMO) keep your mind on high alert even when trying to sleep. This is because the blue light emitted by screens suppresses the production of melatonin, a hormone that regulates sleep. You toss and turn, anticipating the next message, email, or social media update. Each notification jolts you back to wakefulness, disrupting your sleep cycle.

**Turn it around:** Experience the relief of disconnecting from technology by turning off notifications or setting your phone to silent mode at night. Even better, leave the phone outside of your bedroom to resist the temptation to check it before and during sleep. Practice mindfulness techniques to quiet your mind and reduce anxiety about missing out.

## The Sleep Tracker Paradox

While informative, the endless stream of sleep data from wearables and apps can lead to an obsessive focus on achieving 'perfect' sleep. This is because sleep goals, such as a certain number of hours or a specific sleep score, can create unnecessary pressure and anxiety. You find yourself anxious about meeting these goals, ironically making falling asleep harder.

**Turn it around:** Use sleep trackers mindfully, focusing on long-term patterns rather than obsessing over nightly fluctuations. Prioritize consistent sleep routines and a relaxing bedtime environment over trying to "hack" your sleep. Remember, the ultimate goal is to achieve restful sleep, not perfect data.

# About the Author:
## Bibi Ohlsson

Introducing Bibi, a seasoned personal growth advocate, whose unwavering belief in the transformative power of individual strengths has guided her life and career.

Her multicultural background and diverse work-life experiences, from which she draws inspiration, have equipped her with a unique perspective and an innate ability to connect deeply with clients.

With a warm, practical, and highly effective coaching style, Bibi's insightful and action-oriented approach empowers clients to uncover their desired outcomes, work through challenges, and achieve improved well-being and overall life satisfaction.

She's a catalyst for those who seek to live their best lives.

Bibi's global reach and fluency in English and Norwegian allow her to connect with individuals worldwide, ensuring a far-reaching impact.

You can connect with her on
Instagram @evokingexcellence,
visit www.BibiOhlsson.com or email: bibi@evoking-excellence.com to get directly in touch.

# Grimoir of Sleep
*chamber of transformation*

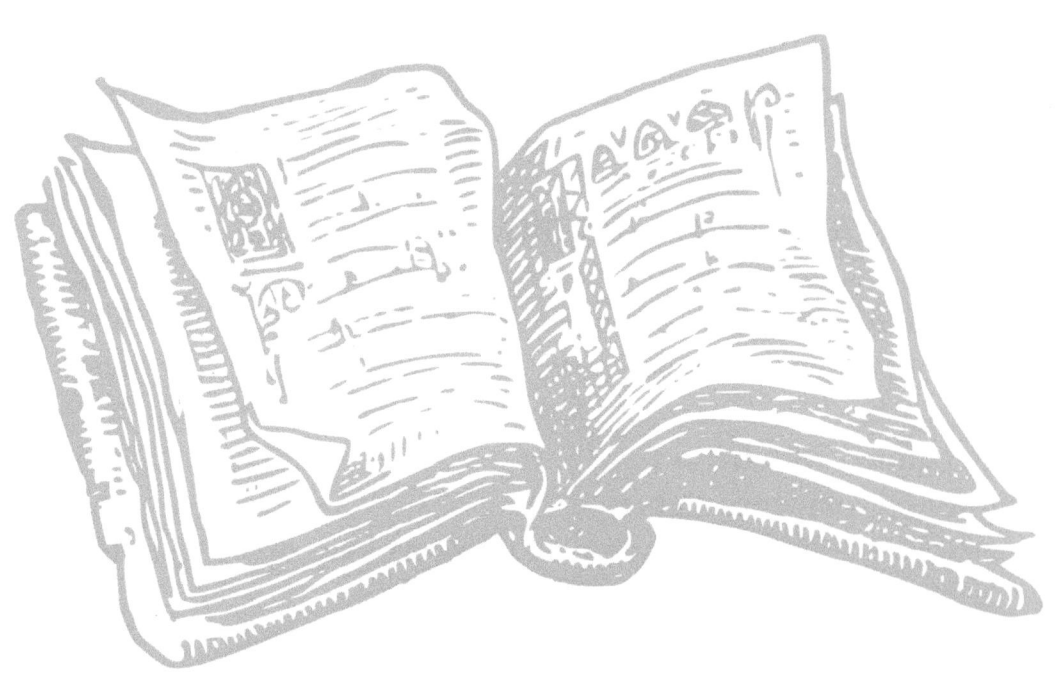

# Emblem of Transformation

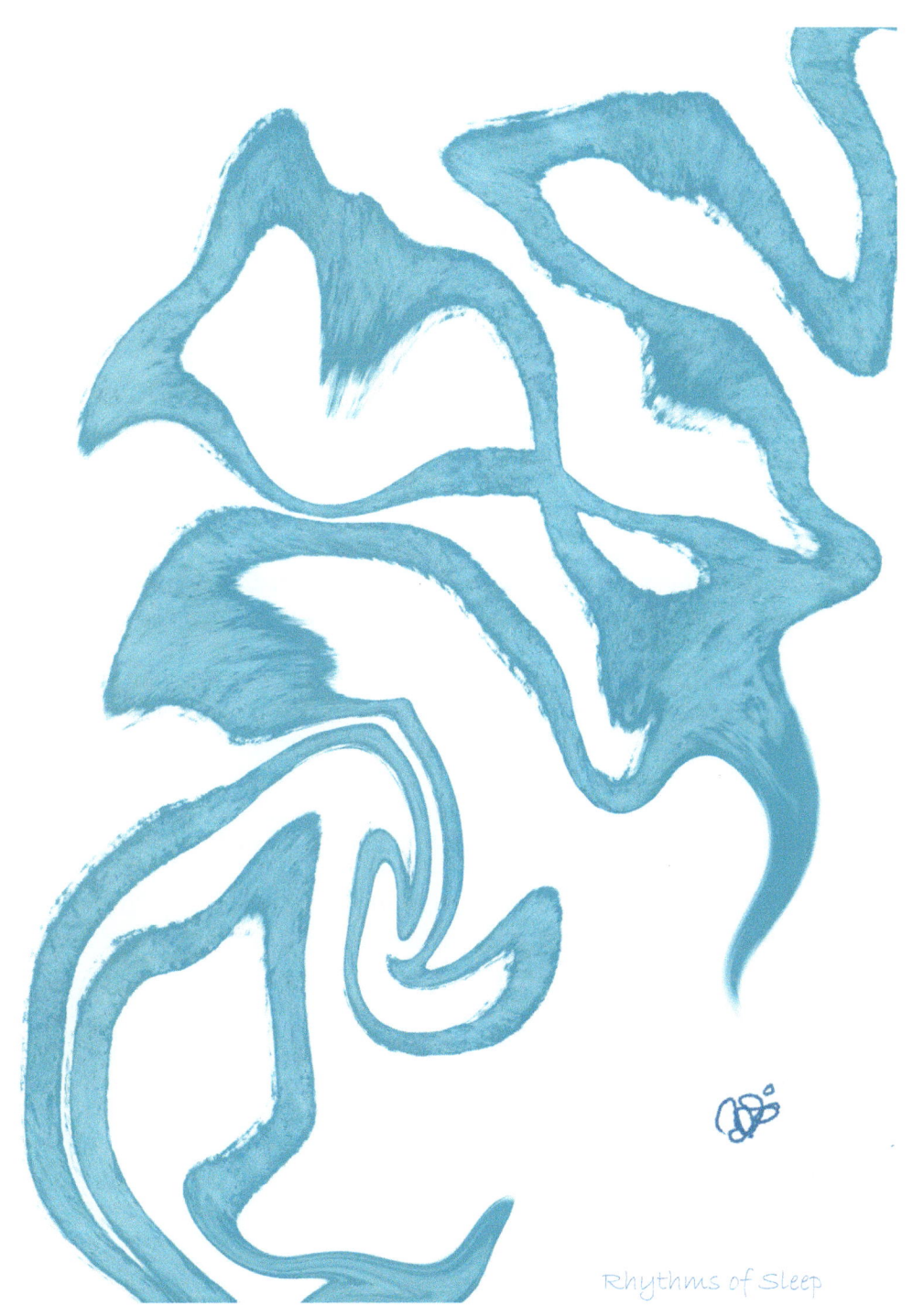

Rhythms of Sleep

*Ready to Awaken Your Sleep?*

*If you see this message, you have likely finished reading my book "Awaken Your Sleep." I hope you found it helpful!*

*I'm reaching out to extend an exclusive invitation to you for a complimentary 30-minute coaching session. This is a unique opportunity to dive deeper into your personal sleep journey and discuss how to apply the book's principles to your unique situation.*

*In this session, we'll explore:*
*Your biggest sleep challenges: What's keeping you up at night?*
*Your sleep goals: What kind of rest and rejuvenation are you seeking?*
*Actionable strategies: How can we tailor the book's teachings to create a personalized sleep plan for you?*

*If you're ready to take the next step in optimizing your sleep simply send me and email and I will get back to you and schedule a mutually convenient time. The coaching session can be conducted via [Zoom/Skype/WhatsApp].*

*I'm excited to hear from you and to support you on your journey to better sleep and a more awakened life! Your potential for improved sleep is limitless, and I'm here to help you unlock it.*

*You can contact me via bibi@evoking-excellence.com, and please provide the code AWAKENYOURSLEEP30 when reaching out.*

*This special offer will remain valid until the end of 2025.*
*Please note that each person can take advantage of this offer for only one session.*